Mindfulness With Yoga

Stress-Free Life And Inner Peace

By

John Francisco

FRANCISCO

Mindfulness With Yoga

This document is geared towards providing exact and reliable information in regards to the topic and issue covered. The publication is sold with the idea that the publisher is not required to render accounting, officially permitted, or otherwise, qualified services. If advice is necessary, legal or professional, a practiced individual in the profession should be ordered.

From a Declaration of Principles which was accepted and approved equally by a Committee of the American Bar Association and a Committee of Publishers and Associations.

The information provided herein is stated to be truthful and consistent, in that any liability, in terms of inattention or otherwise, by any usage or abuse of any policies, processes, or directions contained within is the solitary and utter responsibility of the recipient reader. Under no circumstances will any legal responsibility or blame be held against the publisher for any reparation, damages, or monetary loss due to the information herein, either directly or indirectly.

ACKNOWLEDGMENTS

To Cheryl

Table of Contents:

Introduction

Hello, and welcome to, "Mindfulness With Yoga: Stress-Free Life And Inner Peace." You may be here because you are feeling stressed out in your day to day life. We are here to tell you: YOU ARE NOT ALONE! Did you know that in a 2012 survey, about 20% of American adults stated that they had high levels of stress? It is around 64% of those American adults who said that it was important to manage their stress, while only 37% stated that they could actually manage it.

Stress is something that will happen every now again, as life isn't always a walk in the park. We experience stress from our jobs, our relationships, our families. You may be asking yourself, why must I be stressed all of the time? On a biological standpoint, stress became a part of our human nature to help protect us from physical danger. There is a part of the brain known as the amygdala that sets off this alarm in our brain. When this happens, our body falls into a "fight or flight" response. By doing so, your blood becomes flooded with cortisol and adrenaline and your heart begins racing. When your heart gets going, your blood pressure rises and this is when most of us start to feel STRESSED OUT!

While this response was very important when we were threatened by wildlife while we lived in caves, it can be inconvenient when we get the same response from a little issue at work or a fight with our loved one. Did you know that in Great Britain, stress caused workers to miss 10.4 million working days in one year? Unfortunately, stress can be incredibly debilitating. When we get stressed out, our bodies stop functioning normally. When you become stressed, your body channels energy to the immediate danger and immediately shuts down non-essential systems. Some of these systems are our digestive systems, immune systems, and reproductive systems. After all, why would you need to eat or have sex when you're being chased down by a wolf?

If you're one of the 80% of adults who feel that life is moving too fast to deal with major stress issues, you are not alone. In the following chapters, we will be discussing mindfulness, meditation, and yoga to help you find a way to relax. Whether you want to instantly deal with your stress, or just need a way to unwind at the end of the day, we have got you covered. In our first chapter, we discuss what mindfulness is and how it can help you deal with stress. By learning the "relaxation response," you will become a master of fighting off stress and becoming more cool, calm, and collected in your day to day life.

In our second and third chapter, we go into depth of meditation and yoga practices. You may have heard about the amazing benefits of these exercises, but you never know until you try. We discuss the amazing health benefits and then offer some step by step instructions to get you on your way. No longer will you be in the 50% of adults who have difficulty relaxing when you have a lot to get done. Life is too short to be fighting the demons inside your brain. Now sit back, relax, and enjoy the read.

Chapter One: What is Mindfulness?

You may have come across the concept of mindfulness at some point in your life, but what is it exactly? The term originates from a translation of a Pali-term known as Sati. Sati is an element of Buddhist traditions. In recent popularity in the West. Sati was initiated by a man named Job Kabat-Zinn. Kabat-Zinn is a famous mindfulness meditation teacher and was the founder of a program known as Mindfulness-Based Stress Reduction at the medical center at the University of Massachusetts. We will be learning more about this in a later chapter.

So, what is mindfulness exactly? Some say that it is a psychological process where a person can bring their attention to both internal and external experiences to their mind at the present moment. For most people, they do this through the practice of meditation or yoga. Later in the chapters, will be discussing how you can bring these practices into your daily life. For now, it is important to understand the concept of mindfulness and how it is important for your health.

Mindfulness With Yoga

For some people, accepting what they are feeling is the most difficult concept for them. Unfortunately, this can become a pattern in their day to day life. From first falling into an initial bad experience, then feeling bad about what happens, which leads to feeling bad about feeling bad about a certain situation. As you can tell, this can become a vicious cycle and even worse, be detrimental to one's health! This is where mindfulness comes into play. If you are aware of your thoughts and feelings, you can break the cycle and learn to have a healthier thought process.

You may be thinking, "Well, accepting my feelings just isn't enough." While this may be true, it is certainly an amazing start. By accepting your thoughts, you can accept your feelings. By accepting your feelings, you can step back and take a good hard look at the situation. You can tell yourself that while what you are experiencing may not be ideal, it doesn't mean that you have to be defined by your stress. Instead, mindfulness will teach you that there are healthy ways to accept your thoughts and move on from the moment.

So, where do you begin with mindfulness? Some people have stated that it helps them to locate the emotion within their body. The first step is to realize that the emotion you are feeling is smaller than you are. This way, if you are bigger than the emotion, it means that the stress you are feeling is not everything that you are. By doing this, you can create a space between you as a person and the emotion that you are feeling. By creating space, you may feel like you aren't being suffocated by the problem.

How do you do this? How can you make a stress feeling small? Some have decided to locate the feeling of stress and personify it. For example, try asking yourself some of the following questions: What color is the stress? Does it have a certain texture? Perhaps your feeling is jagged or slimy. Does your stress have a shape? Does it change over a certain amount of time? By giving your stress character, it becomes separate from yourself, therefore, giving you a better grip on the reality of the stress.

According to Kabat-Zinn, his definition of mindfulness is, "...means paying attention in a particular way; on purpose, in the present moment, and nonjudgmentally." His definition highlights the fact that while you practice mindfulness, you must be accepting and always avoid harsh judgments. This gives you the ability to be aware of the experiences surrounding you without pushing the emotions away or even holding them inside. By accepting your emotions, you can be free of them.

While mindfulness involves conscious direction, it important to understand that "mindfulness" and "awareness" are not interchangeable terms. To be mindful, you have to be habitually aware of your feelings. One does not equal the other. If you are aware of a feeling, this does not necessarily mean that you are mindful. Instead, you have to be aware of the situation and then become mindful of it to accept the emotion that you are feeling.

Research studies have found that by being mindful, a large amount of the population have a positive correlation with having a better well-being as well as better health. Mindfulness is also effective to reduce rumination and worry, which have been known to contribute to illnesses such as depression and anxiety. This may be why mindfulness is practiced in psychology to help alleviate both mental and physical conditions of patients. By reducing patients stress through mindfulness, it has been known to help with both anxiety and drug addiction.

For most of us, we are only slightly aware of our thoughts. With this habit, it allows our negative emotions to wander in a very unrestricted way. By having no conscious to bring attention back to the emotion, there is no purpose to the negative emotion we are feeling. This is why we are taught mindfulness to have a purpose to our experiences. By being mindful, you can shape your mind and make your thoughts healthier. You may be asking yourself, what kind of situation would I use this in? For one example, we will be discussing some people's issues with food and the guilty conscious of eating and overeating.

In a health and diet conscious world, some of you may develop an extremely unhealthy relationship with food. While some of us are conscious of what we are putting into our bodies, other may not be. How can we become mindful of our relationship with food? By focusing on our thoughts while we are eating! When an individual is conscious of the process of eating, they can normally notice the sensation of eating such as flavor, color, texture, scent, and more. But, what happens when we are not mindful of what we are eating? Perhaps we are watching the television, talking with friends, reading the newspaper, or simply just thinking about other things. As your mind wanders, you may be not aware of what you are putting into your mouth or how much you are putting into your system. If you are barely aware of the physical sensation of eating, you are probably even less aware of your thoughts and emotions.

Life can be simple, happy, complicated or sad. Life itself is unpredictable, and change is an inevitable factor that goes along with it. Change can hit us in the hardest way possible and leave us on our knees or stumble down. With it, we may seem to lose contact to our inner self and forget the things that make us who we are. When troubles come along the way, we tend to get caught up in the tempest of our emotions and points of view. Ultimately, as we continue our battle to survive, little by little, a piece of us seems to drift astray from what or who we were supposed to be. Until one day, we sit on one corner and feel as if we're lost in the depth of our own thoughts thinking of what ifs in life, re-evaluating our goals and what we have achieved so far. It's fun to say that the bulb of our vivid imagination is always at work and it's doing its trick on our preoccupied selves, turning our frets into a technicolor visions of the future – however, it doesn't work that way. In the end, we have to face reality as it is and deal with the challenges that sprout from anywhere. We have to admit that somehow we failed ourselves, not just in terms of achievements in life but the mere fact that we have deprived ourselves of a healthy or happy way of living.

How can I say so? I've undergone quarter-life crisis and the struggle is definitely real. It even came to a point when I can't even manage to pull myself together and can't even be productive enough at work. Instead, I was unaware that I was already dragging a load of negativity as I continue to sulk. I tried to convince myself that it's ok but my heart says otherwise. Honestly, I can't even think clearly because my thoughts are in complete disarray. It's like I'm trapped in a war within me. Just like what Robert Louis Stevenson wrote in The Strange Case of Dr. Jekyll and Mr. Hyde, "In each of us, two natures are at war – the good and the evil. All our lives the fight goes on between them and one of them must conquer. But in our own hands lies the power to choose – what we want most to be we are." Truly, each one of us has our own chaos within us, but certainly, we have to combat the evil and let the good prevail. Evil comes in different forms and one of which is negativity – a power so cruel that it sucks up all the good and leave you with misery. It was the worst feeling ever. Only you and I have the supremacy over it, and the key is to make the right choice, and I made mine before of which I didn't have any regret. Yes, we had our bad days, but I realized that it's never an excuse to lead a miserable life.

Buddha once said, "Do not dwell in the past, do not dream of the future, concentrate the mind on the present moment." It implies that we should forgive ourselves, accept our once defeat at the shot of life, leave the past behind and just learn from it in order for us to take another chance of moving forward to be better. Just like butterflies, we can allow ourselves to morph beautifully and reveal our true colors. But first, it is important that we find our true inner self.

Though it may be easier to blame or point the finger at something or someone that may have caused the disappointments, in as much as it's harder to accept the truth and move on, still doing the latter breaks the chains that bind us from the haunting experiences of the past.   We have to find that path which will aid us in restoring our self-adoration that once was lost when we were dumbfounded by our failures and mistakes. All we have to do is feel the determination deep within us - a strong will to let go of what hurts us or leaves us melancholy and take a leap of faith towards the bright tomorrow that awaits us. The only person standing between you and your dream is you, and the main element that keeps you from doing what you have to do is FEAR. One way or another you have to conquer it even if it may be tough – just remind yourself that you're as powerful as you think so don't let it take control.

I had my share of less fortunate chapters in my life, and I know you have your own too. I have my fears, but I learned to triumph over it, and then I knew that I'm the only one who could do it; not anyone or anybody else. I found myself better than I was yesterday and all that changed when I made a choice – to be Mindful. I believe that one you could achieve it too! Remember, just will it and it will be yours. You have to stand guard by your goals in rediscovering your true purpose and existence in this world. You may be wondering, how to be mindful? What does being mindful truly mean?

Mindfulness With Yoga

Mindfulness can be described in four simple words: Living in the Moment. It's the condition of appreciating the present situation or moments and living it as it is without having to worry about the past or the distant future. You have to pay attention to what's happening now while you keep your mind rejuvenated to embrace the full experience of the present moments. It is the state of being where your thoughts don't wander off into possibilities of the future or the unknown. Simply, just being caught in the moment and focus on it. It's harder to achieve than it seems, though, but it's not impossible.

Just when I thought about letting my worries devour me and swallow my whole being while the real me is trapped inside, I had an odd dream which I knew meant something. In the dream, a figure was talking to me while I was in a cage made of white sticks; it was telling me to unlock the cage using the key I held on my chest. It just smiled, and I suddenly woke up. I recalled my dream and to my surprise, the key that the figure was trying to point, was actually my gold locket necklace with my picture in it when I was fifteen. Then I remembered that during those years, I started to establish bold life goals and envision myself as I accomplish those goals one at a time. At fifteen I was vigorous, fearless and hopeful. As I pass through the memory lane, I suddenly deciphered the meaning of my dream. The figure I saw was conveying a message to me - to fight my inner demons and let myself be free from it; to rediscover myself and let my wings unfold once again; reveal my true identity that lies inside of me. It might sound bizarre, but in all honesty, it did happen.

It is for this reason that I sought help from a trusted friend, and he suggested that I go through meditation. At first, it sounded a little old school; yet it sounds exactly what I needed at that particular moment. I studied about meditation and mindfulness; ran through several books, journals, online publications/articles and I personally asked my friend to help me. He referred me to his mom's friend, Robert, a 46-year old cheerful lad, who introduced me to the world of Yoga. There are a lot of meditation techniques on how mindfulness can be achieved. The best technique that I've found is Yoga – as based on my experience.

Robert is an active member of a yoga class in our neighborhood, and we shared meaningful conversations about life, I even told him almost everything about me and the whole time I was talking he was actively listening. He shared pieces of his life (which significantly left me in awe) as well as how Yoga helped him live a happy and contented life together with his family. He may stumble upon some challenges along the way, yet he never loses balance or loses his sight on the most important things. His personality oozes with unyielding optimism that's very contagious. When in doubt, he just takes a deep breath and silently drift away into the realm of serenity as his smile curves. Seeing him joyful and lively at his age made me the envy of him but in a good way. He became an inspiration to me and after a while of pondering on things I finally resolved to indulge in Yoga (probably one of the best decisions I ever made).

It may sound old school or traditional, yet after few weeks I already felt the immense change that took place. I felt as if I was touched spiritually – like my soul has been lifted from such heavy burden. I can breathe freely as I close my eyes and feel time pass. Every day I wake up, I feel much more alive, and there's an ample feeling of joy deep in my heart. Better things came into existence, and I never felt more alive.

Given this, I'd like to share relevant points and topics in this book in which I hope could be of great help to others who want to start a new track in the journey of life. It's never too late to let a new chapter of your being commence. This new chapter will offer you insights regarding Yoga, starting off from the very basic information that you have to know. Some may already know a lot, a thing or two and even if you don't have any idea at all, this will serve as your guide if you pursue this activity. Of course, it is unnecessary to learn everything in just one reading; you must take all the time that you need and as much as possible, enjoy yourself while you're reading this (take a sip of coffee if you'd like). If you found lessons that you've grasped, then take it with you and share it with others. It might enlighten them in some ways you'll never know.

In contrast to what most people believe in nowadays, Yoga is more than just an exercise. It's a gradual activity that is beneficial to your mind, body, and spirit. It takes time but it's an investment that will truly reward you with impressive results. Also, included in this book are the essentials that you'll be needing before you start Yoga and tips about routines as well as diet plans that work best for a tip-top shape body.

Mindfulness With Yoga

You'll obtain benefits that Yoga could provide you, and if you're conscious about keeping a fit body and right weight, you'll find significant how-to information here. Also, best poses that are effective in losing weight can be found in this book. Every pose signifies a profound sense which you will come to understand more as you read along. Furthermore, you'll encounter formulas to fulfill happier and healthier life and how Yoga can greatly affect your standpoint or outlook in life. There's much more to learn and discover, and this book will walk you through to what lies ahead of you.

Yoga is just a piece of the puzzle, but once you have unraveled the secrets you hold within you, things will be exciting, and it will put things into perspective. Just don't forget to embody the teachings of Yoga – it's more than just a physical routine but a healing therapy. Once your wounds heal and scars fade away, ultimately you'll become a stronger person who will never back down from anything that life throws at you.

The main question is; how do I bring the practice of mindfulness into my daily life? The answer is simple: purpose. To be mindful of your emotions, you must be able to find purposefulness in your actions and experiences. You must actively shape your mind in order to be mindful, and we are here to show you a few different ways to get started.

Be in the Moment

We've all been in the moment when we let our emotions get the best of us. Whether you allow yourself to wallow in self-pity after a bad break up, get extremely pissed when you are stuck in traffic, fall into a depression, feel like seeking revenge, or even just simply are craving a chocolate chip cookie like crazy, these are ALL examples of allowing the mind to wander with negative thoughts and emotions. When we indulge our brains with these thoughts, you are reinforcing your emotions and causing self-harm to your being. The thing is, most of these emotions take place in the past and the future. You are allowing these emotions that no longer exist, bother you in the present. What we must remember is that the future is a fantasy until the moment arrives. The only moment that we can experience is the here and the now. Unfortunately, it is a moment that most of us tend to avoid because we are too concerned about the time surrounding the present. This is where mindfulness comes into play.

When you become mindful of your experiences and your emotions, you pull your conscious into the present. Now, this doesn't mean that you never have to think about the past or the future, but it does mean that we must be mindful of thinking about the past and the future. When you direct your awareness from thoughts of a different time and anchor yourself into the present moment, you can decrease negative emotions in your present life. By doing so, you can fall into a certain calmness and allow yourself to grow from these emotions.

Allow Yourself to be Non-judgmental

As we mentioned earlier, mindfulness is about living in the present moment and being as non-judgmental as possible. While in practice, mindfulness is a non-reactive state. By doing so, you must remind yourself that a certain experience isn't good or bad. Instead, you must become aware of the experience, take notice of them, and then let it go. By being mindful, this allows you not to get upset over an experience you do not want to be a part of. By being mindful, you accept the moment as it arrives and then allow it to pass and cease to exist. This way, it cannot negatively affect you. Whether it is pleasant or painful, you must treat each experience in the same manner.

Fixing your Thoughts and Conscious

Now that you understand that you must be mindful of your experiences, the question is, how can you fix your thoughts? Remember that while there are both pleasant and unpleasant experiences, you must remember to keep a certain stillness and a balance of your mind. You can do this by developing an acceptance in a friendly curiosity. The main purpose of mindfulness is to have this attitude of acceptance. By doing so, you get your thoughts away from pushing the experience away or clinging onto it. The first step of moving on from the moment is to fully recognize where you are, how you are feeling, and how to move on. For practice, try telling yourself: "It's okay," "Let me feel this," and "It is okay to feel this way." By repeating this to yourself, you are averting the negative emotions and creating a creative response to the situation. By telling yourself that the emotions you are feeling are acceptable, you can break out of the vicious cycle of feeling bad as we had mentioned earlier.

It is important to realize that to be healthy and mindful, you must have the ability to stand back from your thoughts and emotions whether they be negative or positive. You must consciously realize that the thoughts in your mind are not your true reality. When your thoughts begin to race, allow them to stream and then let them go. Remember that thoughts only occur if we put our time and energy into them. If you want to let go of the negative energy, you simply stop them from being created and create a space of freedom for yourself.

While it may seem complicated, letting go of your thoughts can be made easy. For some people, all it takes is simply labeling your thoughts as useful. Often, you may notice that you are thinking to yourself. When you find yourself deep in thought, try whispering the word "thinking" to yourself so that you can name your experience and then let it go and move on from the moment. If this doesn't work for you, try adapting to a skeptical attitude of your thoughts. At times, thoughts can either bring us down or empower us. Instead of instantly believing your thoughts, question your beliefs and then become aware that what you were thinking is only a thought. By doing so, this will also allow you to move on from the moment.

Some of us may need a bit more than just keeping our thoughts in and out of our brain. In the next few chapters, we will be discussing the benefits of both meditation and yoga for mindfulness. By bringing these practices into your daily life, you can become mindful and reap the benefits of practicing these relaxing exercises. We offer you the details of the practice and a step-by-step guide to getting you started. Our main goal is to help teach you how to become relaxed and live a healthier life. We hope you are enjoying the read so far. Stick around for the next chapter of Meditation for Mindfulness.

Chapter Two: Meditation for Mindfulness

You have probably heard the term "meditation" before and how it helps most people relax and calm down. So, how is it related to mindfulness? The practice of mindfulness meditation is unique because it is done to help you become aware of each moment that passes. By being aware of the true moment, it steers you away from getting you to be different and be who you are as an individual. By doing so, it can help us recognize our wisdom and in return, teach us to stop our thoughts from torturing us. By being aware of our feelings, we can turn our thoughts away from discomfort, pain, and bad experiences and realize that these moments are an inevitable experience of being alive.

For most individuals, mindfulness meditation is practiced while sitting down. While in the sitting position, this can take place cross-legged while on a cushion or even while sitting on a chair but remember to have your back straight. The sitting practice allows the opportunity to be present with yourself, in the moment, exactly as you are. While sitting, you will want to place your attention to the movement of your abdomen as you breathe in and out. You want your awareness to be only on your breath, bringing the air in and out of your nostrils. Of course, your thoughts may begin to wander as you breathe, but just consciously remind yourself that you are thinking something, accept the thought, and then return to focus on your breath. One would think something so simple couldn't do much, but as we will be learning in this chapter, mindfulness meditation has many incredible benefits.

Before we get into the actual practice of mindfulness meditation, we want to take a moment to remind you that mindfulness is all about having nonjudgmental attention to your experience. As a beginner, you may become frustrated and find meditation more difficult than you expected. Remind yourself that this is okay! Instead of struggling with the experience, we wish for you to practice dealing with the situation. If you catch onto the practice, remember to be mindful of the experience if it is pleasant as well. Many people have a hard time staying in the present if they are happy. Often, people will begin to worry more about making the feeling last or grasping onto the situation to keep it from fading away. As you practice, accept the moment of happiness and then let it go.

If this will be your first time meditating, do not worry if you cannot stop thoughts from passing through your mind. Most people feel that their thoughts should be completely stopped and that they just need to rest their minds to find peace. Remember that having thoughts is a normal concept that is supposed to happen! Having thoughts should not be thought of as a negative consequence. Instead, accept the thoughts and allow them to pass. When you notice yourself becoming distracted, simply accept the thought and then bring your attention back to meditation. With more practice, you will find yourself increasing your ability to concentrate and focus on your breathing. It is then that you will have conquered mindfulness. For now, we will be teaching you the basic concepts of meditation so that you can get started on your path of consciousness and relaxation.

Interestingly enough, studies have shown that for those who use mindfulness meditation, there have been effects on the attention regulation, emotional regulation as well as body awareness. The studies also showed that the practice leads to a more coherent and a healthier sense of self when used to study authenticity, compassion, character, self-acceptance and even responsibility. If this isn't reason enough to convince you to practice mindfulness meditation, did you know that the practice has been known to actually change your brain?

Your Brain on Meditation

While there are many amazing benefits of meditation, it is specifically beneficial for your emotional well-being, your brain, and your body. Those who practice were less likely to be impulsive, they worry less, they had a heightened self-esteem and even were more likely to build positive social connections. These individuals also had an improved immune system, higher energy levels, and a reduced blood pressure. We will be breaking down the benefits between the brain, the body, and your well-being just to convince you that mindfulness meditation can be an amazing added benefit to your daily routine!

Depression and Anxiety

Studies have shown that mindfulness helps decrease depression in both schools and mothers to be! In a study done in Belgium, around 400 students in five different middle schools were placed in a mindfulness program. After six months, they reported that that had reduced stress, anxiety, and depression. According to another study, the scientist concluded that mindfulness meditation could be just as effective as antidepressant drug therapy. For those of you who are wildly against the heavy medicated society we live in, meditation may be the proper cure for your emotions.

In a different study held for pregnant woman, the women participated in a ten-week mindfulness yoga class where the results showed that there was a reduction in depression. Along with a lowered depression symptom, these mothers also had a more intense bonding session with their babies while they were still in the womb! This may be because meditation truly helps people regulate their mood as well as their anxiety disorders.

Focus, Attention, and Decision-Making

If you ever feel like you have a hard time concentrating, you are not alone! In a study done at the University of California, they found that their subjects had an easier time keeping focus on repetitive and boring tasks after short meditation training. In some cases, they even did so much as ten times better than the control group. The people who practiced meditation did a better job on information tasks, even when they were assigned a stressful deadline.

Studies also found that those who practiced meditation for a long time had larger amounts of gyrification in their brain. In simple terms, this is a part of the brain that allows your brain to process information faster. It is this fold on the cortex that allows us to make decisions, form memories, and improves your attention!

Speaking of paying attention, did you know that meditation has also been known to help manage ADHD symptoms? In a study done with 50 adults who had ADHD, the group who participated in MBCT (we cover this later) or Mindfulness-based cognitive therapy, showed reduced impulse and reduced hyperactivity.

Benefits of Meditation and Your Body

Some of us get worked up because of the thoughts in our mind, but what about the worries about our body? It is part of the conscious to realize that we all have a limited time on this earth, but what about taking care of the body you were given? While some of us may suffer from certain illnesses, meditation has been known to help improve health and reduce the risk of certain diseases. While there are numerous amazing benefits for the body when one meditates, we will just touch on a few of the benefits that are important.

Reduced Risk-Heart Disease and Stroke

In a study done in 2012, a group of high-risk individuals took a class of meditation. Over the five years following this class, the participants were found to have a 48% reduction in the risk of heart attack and stroke. This was classified when these individuals were found to have a lower blood pressure and a lowered psychosocial stress factors. This may be because meditation has been known to affect the genes that can control both stress and immunity. Those who participated in meditation had improvements in their immune system and had a higher resilience to stressful situations.

When you are less stressed, this means that your blood pressure will be lower. In a study done following the technique of "relaxation response," the patients had a drop in blood pressure after participating in 3 months of mediation. By being more relaxed, they needed less medication. When one is relaxed, this allows for nitric oxide to form in the body, opening up the blood vessels.

Reduces Risk- Premature Death and Alzheimer's

In a study published in *the Brain, Behavior, and Immunity* journal, the results stated that 30 minutes of meditation per day could reduce the risk of heart disease, depression, Alzheimer's and premature death. Just imagine taking such a short amount of time out of your day, to improve the quality and quantity of your life!

Yes, you read that correctly. Some scientists believe that meditation may indeed help you live longer. An important aspect of this is a little thing called Telomeres. These are a part of the human cell in which affects how our cells age. By reducing stress arousal and increasing a positive state of mind, this may help promote telomere maintenance.

With all of these amazing benefits, why wouldn't you start meditating? If you wish to learn how you can start meditating yourself, continue reading below.

Getting Started with Meditation

Before we begin with instructions on meditation, you must first be aware that there are three basic aspects of meditation. These include: body, breath, and thoughts. We will be going into depth on each of these steps to better prepare yourself for meditation. If you are a beginner, do not worry about getting it absolutely perfect the first time. Meditation is different for everyone. While some of you will be more comfortable on the floor, others will prefer being in a chair. Eventually, you will find your own manner of meditation in a way that will make you relaxed and happy. While these are just suggestions from popular practices, we invite you to find your twist on meditation. All you need is a little space, a little time, and a little thought and you will be well on your way to mindfulness meditation.

Body

The very first aspect of meditation is having a focus on your body. You will want to begin your practice by setting up an environment where you feel safe, comfortable, and relaxed. For some people, meditation is used to prepare oneself to work with others. In this is the concept, you will want to practice with your eyes open. You will want to put your focus on an item in front of you. For most people, they will choose just a corner or a small spot in their home to set up their quiet space. It is very rare for people to choose an entire room as the subject of their focus. Once you have picked your little spot, it will be time to choose your seat.

As we had mentioned earlier, each practice session will be unique in its own way. The main function is that you are comfortable. While some people choose to sit on a cushion on the floor, others decide to use a chair. It is suggested that if you are to choose a cushion for the ground, perhaps invest in one that was designed for meditation such as a gomden or a zafu. If you are a beginner, try folding a blanket or using a low bench. Before you begin your practice, you simply want to make sure that your seat is stable, so you aren't distracted by wiggling around.

If you do decide on a chair, be sure that the one you choose does not tilt in the back and has a flat seat. While in the chair, you will want to make sure that your feet touch the ground. If you are on the shorter side, perhaps try putting a bench on the floor to rest your feet. While having your legs dangling as first may be comfortable, it may become uncomfortable over time and draw you away from your meditation practice. For those of you who may be taller, be sure that your hips are higher than your knees. If you fail to do this, your back may begin to start hurting, drawing you away from the practice again.

For your body, the ideal posture is to be sitting upright but not to the point where you are rigid. Your posture should reflect your sanity. Ideally, you would be dignified but not stiff. While sitting, try keeping your back straight while having a curve on the lower back. Try imagining that your spine is a tree that you need to lean against. Your body will take natural form for instant comfort.

The same posture stands if you are sitting on a cushion. While sitting, you will want to make sure that your legs are crossed comfortably in front of you. While some meditators have been known to have an uncomfortable looking posture, there is absolutely no reason to contort yourself to be any more "professional." Think of yourself in your childhood and simply cross your legs one over another. You may notice that your hips become higher than your knees. If you wish, try adding height to your seat by sitting on another blanket. You will want to choose whichever works best for you as an individual.

Once you are sitting in a comfortable position, whether it be on a cushion or a chair, you will then bring your hands to a relaxing rest on your thighs while facing down. Your eyes should be somewhat open while holding your gaze about six feet away from you on the floor. If you are sitting on the ground, feel free to gaze at the wall in front of you. Your eyes are not extremely important in this practice. Instead, your eyes should not be tightly focused. Just look ahead and allow your eyes to rest where they are set.

When you are comfortable, sit in this position in your environment for just a few minutes. You may find your attention wandering away. If this happens, you will just want to bring your body back to your environment as gently as possible. Remember, as a beginner, your mind will wander, but this is part of the mindfulness meditation. Be aware that your thoughts are going, become conscious of the situation in a nonjudgmental manner and then bring your body back to the environment you have created. Remember to keep your front open, your back strong, and you are ready for the next step of mindfulness meditation.

Breath

Now that we have you sitting on your cushion or your chair, becoming aware of your thoughts and your environment, it's time to start focusing on the next part: your breath. While sitting, begin to practice bringing attention to your breath. As you breathe, feel it come into your body and feel again as it leaves your body. The same as sitting, there is no special technique to breathing. For mindfulness meditation, we want you to be intrigued by how you are and how you respond when you consciously think about your breathing. You will want to accept the fact that you are controlling your breathing lightly. If you are a beginner, remember not to get caught up on breathing normally. When you are focused on the action, it can be hard to be natural on purpose. Remember that we are all different and allow your breath to be as it is. As time goes on, you will find your breathing becoming more normal and less of a conscious task.

We want to remind you that the point of the

practice isn't to get it right or perfect. The idea behind mindfulness meditation is to give you an idea of channeling your thoughts. In this case, we want you to focus your attention on breathing naturally. You can do so by sitting for a few minutes and focusing on your breathing and your breathing alone. The same as getting acclimated to your environment, learn the simple process of your breathing. Feel as the air slips in and out of your nostrils. Feel how such a seemingly simple task is keeping your whole body functioning properly. While only some of your conscious should be focused on your breathing, remember to bring the rest of your attention back to your body and back to your environment. You should be focused on all three (breathing, body, and environment). Accept your thoughts, be aware of them, and then let them go as you bring your attention back to your breathing. Once you have mastered this, you are ready for the third part of mindfulness meditation.

Thoughts

As we mentioned earlier, thoughts are a normal part of our existence. While some thoughts are great, others may be more distracting. We all have thoughts like plans for our future, certain fantasies, and even memories of our past. For most of us, one leads to another, and there is no gap for us to be able to catch our breath. As you sit and practice, just be aware of your thoughts. The point of mindfulness meditation is not about getting yourself to stop thinking. When you find yourself lost in thought while meditating, take notice that it is happening. You will want to remind yourself that you are who you are and that you do not need to change yourself. Do not become discouraged when thoughts overcome your mind. Simply accept, and move on.

To start out mindfulness meditation, try starting out with short periods of about 10 minutes a day. Remember that the more you practice, the easier it will be to focus on your breathing. Start out with the first step before adding the second and finally the third. Once you have practiced enough, you will be fully aware of your thoughts, your feelings, and even your actions. For now, remember that it is acceptable to be a beginner and that you will not be an expert straight out of the gates. In the end, you will be lucky enough to feel the health benefits of meditation.

Chapter Three: Yoga and Mindfulness

If meditation isn't up your alley, perhaps yoga is! Yoga is one of the best ways to fight the stress in your life, all while getting the benefits of getting in shape and leading a healthier life. The practice of yoga is a mind and body exercise that combines the controlled breathing, physical poses, and meditation all in one. The best part is, yoga is for people of all different shapes and ages. To some, Yoga is a complementary health approach that brings the physical and the mental being together. The main concept is to achieve peacefulness and in return, you will be able to handle your stress and anxiety in a healthy manner.

As mentioned earlier, yoga can be for just about everyone. There are several forms of yoga, one example being hatha yoga. This form of yoga is common among beginners as it has a slow pace and easy movements. Hatha yoga is also a great choice for those looking for an exercise that can help manage stress. At the end of the day, it is about a personal preference for what works for you.

The practice of yoga is composed of three

different techniques. The first being what yoga is most commonly known for, poses. These yoga poses are also known as postures. While in poses, yoga is made of a series of movements in which were designed to help increase both strength and flexibility. If you are a beginner, these poses can range from lying on the floor, all the way to more difficult positions that can test your physical limits.

Just like meditation, one of the main focuses of yoga is on breathing. While coming in and out of poses, you must learn how to control your breathing. By concentrating on your breath, it can help both control your body as well as quiet your mind. By silencing your thoughts, you may find yourself completely relaxed. Meditation is the third and last aspect of yoga. By being aware of the present moment without judgment, you can learn how to relax and enjoy the moment that is surrounding you.

Yoga: What You Need To Know First

Did you know that Yoga originated in India? This is just one of the many things you need to know about Yoga. There's a lot more to discover.

1. A Peek From The Past: Brief History of Yoga

Five thousand years ago, Ancient Yogis (practitioners of yoga) from India believed that the human body should be appreciated and respected for it is the reflection of man's growth and work. It is with this body of wisdom that gave birth to Yoga. The term Yoga was taken from the Sanskrit word "Yuj" which means "to unite or integrate." The main goal of this practice is to unify the mind, body, and soul which creates harmony and discipline.

Yoga is divided into four distinct periods: the Vedic Period, Pre-Classical Period, Classical Period, and Post-Classical Period.

Yoga was developed during the Vedic Period, a time when Vedas (sacred Brahmanism scripture) were at its prevalent existence. It is known to contain the oldest Yogic teachings called Vedic Yoga, which attempts to transcend the limitations of the human mind through rituals and ceremonies.

In the search for life in divine harmony, Vedic people searched for teachings not only from Vedic Yogis but also from individuals whose rigorous spiritual practice grants them the ability to see the ultimate reality. These individuals were known as Rishis. Some Yogis and Rishis even lived in total seclusion deep within the forests to achieve their ultimate goal of understanding the world.

Despite its origin, Hinduism isn't the only one that shares characteristics with Yoga but Buddhism as well. When Buddha started his teachings of Buddhism way back 6th century B.C, meditation has been the main focus and Yoga evolved from then on. Siddharta Gautama, at the age of 35, was the first Buddhist to study this practice and accomplished self-enlightenment. Aside from that, the creation of Upanishads defined the Pre-Classical Period through series of Hindu sacred scriptures which expounded the Vedas.

During the Classical Period, another evolution of Yoga was recorded. Around 2nd century, Patanjali wrote Yoga Sutra, which is composed of 95 aphorisms or sutras (thread in Sanskrit literature). It presented the Eightfold Path of Yoga (also called Eight Limbs of Classical Yoga) which is considered the fundamental handbook on the system of yoga. Here are the Eight Limbs of Patanjali: **Dharana,** concentration; **Yama,** social restraints or ethical values; **Niyama**, personal observance of purity, tolerance, and study; **Asanas** or physical exercises; **Pranayama**, meaning breath control or regulation; **Pratyahara,** the spirit withdrawal in preparation for meditation; **Dhyana,** which means Meditation; and **Samadhi,** which means ecstasy. These were suggestions for a better life.

Lastly, the Post-Classical Period or also known as Modern Yoga, unlike the other three periods, is focused on being mindfulness. Its teachings attempt to let the person appreciate and live at the moment. During this period, Yoga Guru Swami Sivananda created the five basic principles of Yoga, namely: **Proper diet; Correct breathing; Proper relaxation; Proper exercise; Positive thinking and Meditation.**

2.   What are the Different Types of Yoga?

There are six most common types of Yoga and four main paths of Yoga, namely: Karma, Bhakti, Raja, and Jnana. Each one has its distinct characteristics as well as the level of difficulty. Since there are a lot to choose from, you may have a tough time in selecting the best practice that would suit you best, but eventually, you'll find one that you like.

- **Hatha Yoga** – it is regarded as the therapeutic branch of yoga and the most popular among them all. This practice concentrates on gentle postures, movements, and breathing control. The main focus of this branch is to calm the body and mind in preparation for meditation to achieve total wellness.

- **Bhakti Yoga** – derived from the word Bhakti, which means "devotion." In this branch, you're required to have a strong sense of faith and surrender yourself to God. It is considered to be the most direct method to achieve oneness in everything.

- **Karma Yoga** – this branch of yoga is also known as the "yoga of action." It helps achieve divine harmony through selfless actions without expecting anything in return, instead, offering them up to the Almighty. By doing so, you'll learn to liberate yourself from the confines of your ego.
- **Kundalini Yoga** – Kundalini originated from one of the oldest forms of spirituality, the tantra yoga. Kundalini Yoga is a combination of spiritual and physical practices which surrounds the area of the lower spine. Its goal is to build physical strength

while increasing consciousness. However, this practice is usually performed only by those who are well advanced in the practices of spirituality.

- **Raja Yoga** – translated from the Sanskrit, means Royal Union. It is described as the royal path to achieving the unity of mind, body, and spirit. This branch follows the teachings of the Eight Limbs Path (the ones we mentioned in the classical period of Yoga): Yama, Niyama, Asana, Pranayama, Pratyahara, Dharana- concentration, Dhyana- meditation, and Samadhi.

- **Jnana Yoga** – also known as "The Yoga of Wisdom," is considered to be the most difficult among the four main paths of Yoga (Karma, Bhakti, Raja, Jnana). This branch requires the extreme strength of will and intellect in search of true knowledge. It utilizes intellect to realize that our true self is beyond and behind our mind.

Note: If you wish to determine further which branch or type of Yoga would work best for you, you should conduct deeper research to gain a better understanding. All of these types are equally unique and don't have to compare which one is better than the other because the truth is, there's no such thing as "better style". Besides, there is no right or wrong choice of practice. You just have to make sure that you take your time and consider your personality as well as individuality when you make your choice.

3. Debunking Common Yoga Misconceptions

Yoga is not just an exercise – it's way more than that. Probably, you have heard a few things that people have been saying about it which makes you wonder whether to believe it or not. Through the years, facts have been discovered along with it are common misconceptions about Yoga, but there are no absolutes. Change is bound to happen every day. To help you sort things out, here's the list of fallacies people can't help but talk about:

- **Typical Stereotyping -** First of all, Yoga isn't only good for skinny, young or single people. I know a lot of people complaining about how their physical looks make them unfit for it. It's like saying that plus size people can't be models, or black people can't be great leaders. We have to stop this mentality. Yoga is a practice that knows no size, gender, age, race or social status – whoever and whatever you are, you can do it. It benefits anyone who chooses to live by its teachings and techniques. The only requirement here is an open and determined mind.

- **Religion -** The first time I entered a yoga studio, I saw a Hindu statue and I noticed the chants as well. Some people may have experienced it as well and thinking that Yoga, as history wrote, have Hinduism and Buddhism beliefs and traditions, it can't be helped that thought about religion will be brought up. Nevertheless, Yoga is not a religion and does not create any conflicts with it at all. It's just like moving meditation in which you are spiritually involved in finding harmony within your mind and body. Teachings and philosophies from the Sanskrit and Brahman scriptures have helped change a lot of lives, including Christians, Muslims, Jews and a whole lot more. It shouldn't be a topic for a non-sense argument.

- **Yoga is For Physical Fitness -** In modern yoga, one of the principles include exercise, and this is what most people seem to get wrong. Aside from its health benefits, Yoga offers mindfulness and a spiritual healing that can help fulfill a happy life. Unlike other exercises like Zumba, movements in

Yoga go in rhythm creating a harmony with the mind and body. It serves as the path to achieving self-enlightenment and awareness.

- **Yoga is Easy and Exclusive For Girls -** This is a big NO! Yoga has gentle poses and movements, but it doesn't mean that it is easy, and nobody said it is only for girls. Let's take Karma Yoga for example. It includes intense routines that will even leave the boys (including me) sweating. Again, Yoga is not gender specific.

- **Only Vegetarians Are Allowed -** There is no solid law that denies meat-eaters the right to attend Yoga classes. Even in the Sanskrit or Hindu scriptures, it was never mentioned that to fulfill divine purpose one shall not eat meat! Preferring meat for consumption was never the basis of accepting people to participate in Yoga. Nobody said that you have to follow every Yoga practice. If you want to eat meat, then go ahead and eat meat. Nobody will stop you.

4. The Yoga Checklist: Essentials that You Need To Have

In everything you do, you always have to be

prepared. Before getting yourself into the world of Yoga, you will need few things to get you started. The question is, what are the things you need? Here is a list of essentials for you to check and follow.

- **Yoga Outfits -** This should be the first thing on your list. Here's the thing, though, Yoga outfits are not the same as gym outfits. In order for you to move freely while you are enjoying Yoga, choose a snug-fitting wear. Tops, shorts, pants or capris can be worn during Yoga class but make sure that the material is light. Avoid any unnecessary items like jewelry, socks, leg warmers and scarves.

- **Yoga Mat -** It is important to ensure a Yoga Mat before joining classes and quality should be taken into consideration. You can technically buy these mats anywhere, but you have to be very keen on buying one. Here are few points to remember: Check the Material – you can opt for rubber or non-stick mats to give you a better grip, or if you're prone to sweating, it's best to invest in organic mat due to the Texture and thickness. The texture will allow for more traction and avoid slipping, plus, a decent amount of cushion helps maintain better balance.

- **Yoga Bag -** Certainly, you would want to keep all your things in one place and avoid lost stuff. A Yoga Bag allows you to keep your belongings in check for easier access. Select a bag that's just appropriate for your things and comfortable for you to carry along.

- **Meditation cushions -** A Meditation Cushion lets you optimally do your routines in a relaxed but alert mode. Most of the time, you will not be aware of how long you have already been sitting or doing a certain pose. Given this, to avoid sore bottom or body parts, it is important that you include meditation cushions as essentials. The comfier, the better.

- **Foam blocks -** This is one of the most commonly used props in yoga class. Foam blocks allow you to deepen and enjoy practice more. It has four basic functions: for flexibility, to provide support, for balance, for longer and comfortable position. It is available in various shapes, sizes, and design. The choice is up to you.

- **Yoga Straps -** Just like foam blocks, yoga straps are beneficial not only to beginners but also to experienced yogis. It can help you with alignment, posture, and support while doing this practice. It allows stretching to be more enjoyable and effective while maintaining the structural alignment of your body, especially in some poses.

Note: Aside from the above-mentioned essentials, you may need a few more items along the way. Or if your Yoga teacher requires additional props such as yoga balls, hand pumps, or yoga straps, then go ahead and get them. If you're doing Yoga at home, prioritize safety.

Why Should I Practice Yoga?

Of course, Yoga offers many benefits other than just helping you relax. If you aren't convinced yet that yoga could be the right choice for you, here are ten reasons you should consider Yoga. If you feel Yoga is something you'd like to try, you can skip ahead to read our step by step guide to get you started on your Yoga journey.

1. **Convenience**
Did you know that Yoga is a $27 billion industry? In recent years, the practice is becoming more and more popular! No matter where you may be

living, there is sure to be a yoga studio near you, and there are more popping up every week. If you happen to live in the country that does not offer yoga, don't sweat! All you need is some space and a mat. Try practicing yoga in your living room, your backyard, or even the park! Be sure to make some time to practice yoga today.

2. **Growing Strong**
   Some yoga poses are more difficult than they look. By holding certain poses and moving through poses such as sun salutations, it can help you grow some muscle! According to studies, yoga practice has been linked to a greater dead-life strength. If you are trying to gain muscle, perhaps it is time to fit some yoga practice into your schedule.

3. **Flying Solo**
   As we mentioned earlier, sometimes yoga can be held in studios. However, the practice itself is usually an individual practice. While friends may surround you, it is important that you take some of this time alone so that you can reflect, see, and evaluate your life. Sometimes, it may even be your friends that are the source of your stress. If this is the case, spend some deep thinking time in the

Child's Pose to allow you to gather your thoughts, come to terms, and then let your thoughts go.

4. **Never Get Bored**
   Although we only mentioned hatha yoga earlier, there are several different types depending on what you are looking for in a yoga practice. For example, if you are looking to get into shape and maybe even break a sweat? You can try Vinyasa yoga. If you're looking for a more relaxing type of yoga where you can just breathe and stretch, try Hatha or Yin yoga. Luckily, there is a type of yoga out there for just about anyone. If you're feeling adventurous, why not explore a few different types?

5. **Let's get Flexible**
   According to some studies, it only takes about six weeks of yoga practice to increase your flexibility. By practicing yoga, you may be prompted to try out new poses, meditative thoughts, or even breathing styles. Yoga can flex not only your body but also your mind. When was the last time you were flexible? The stretching is good for your body and good for your mental health.

6. **Reducing Anxiety**

Later in this chapter, we will be discussing the amazing benefits of yoga. Were you aware that after just 12 weeks of yoga, people reported to have a reduces anxiety level? People who stress less normally smile more. The exercise that comes from yoga can help boost happy chemicals to your brain and in return, can improve your mood. This is why some doctors have turned to yoga as a suggestion for their patients that may suffer from depression.

7. **Challenge Yourself**
   One of the best parts of yoga is that you do not need to be an expert. Every practice of yoga will be your own. The only person that you may be competing against is yourself. When you begin to practice, see if you can increase your concentration, stretch a little deeper into your pose or hold onto the position a little longer. By challenging yourself, you will be able to feel yourself grow and change over time.

8. **Brain Power**
   If you find yourself stressed out more during your day to day tasks, it may be time to roll out your mat and clear your mind. According to some studies, yoga can increase brain function in as

little as 20 minutes after you finish. By clearing your mind, this can lead to an improved memory and may help maintain some of your focus. As we mentioned earlier, you do not need a lot of space to practice yoga. If you find yourself stressing and falling behind at work, it could be time for some yoga to help give you a leg up at work!

9. **QUIET!**

Let's face it. There are those moments every now again that we just wish for a little bit of quiet time. Whether you need to get away from your chatty husband, your screaming children, or you're just bored of listening to the same five songs on the radio, try getting yourself into a traditional yoga class. Here, you can soak in the silence and truly relax your mind. Sometimes all it takes is a little peace and quiet to help you relax and get in touch with your breath.

10. **Get Social**

Remember how we said that yoga is gaining popularity? Get out there and make some friends! Sure, we all need a little quiet time, but we also need to surround ourselves with people who can understand our story. By finding fellow yoga people, you can all relax and get in touch with your inner self through yoga. Having an exercise partner may even push you to push yourself. There is no better way to motivate yourself and others by doing what you love. After all, being around people who practice yoga may help you relax even further when you are surrounded by people immersed in yoga.

Yoga and Health Benefits

While the last section was pretty convincing in itself, did you know that yoga also offers numerous health benefits? While a big majority of people believe that yoga is just a fad at the gym, in fact, yoga has been practiced for centuries and can connect the mind, the body, and the spirit through a number of poses. Below, is a list some of the amazing benefits you could be getting through practicing yoga yourself!

Exercise Benefits

Muscle Tone: Who isn't looking for some beautiful muscle tone? Those who consistently practice yoga have reported better muscle tone in their body.

Joint Range: There was a recent study done at the School of Medicine at the University of Pennsylvania that stated that for those who practiced yoga, they gained a better joint range of motion. If you're looking for more flexibility, yoga could be a top choice for you.

Dexterity: As we mentioned earlier, yoga can connect the mind and body. Through the practice of yoga, you could see yourself gaining some grace and some skill.

Non-competitive: You now know that yoga is a solo sport. Yoga removes any form of competition from its exercise regimen. Instead, the nature of yoga is both introspective and self-building to help you grow as an individual.

Endurance: Yoga can be an entire body workout. For those who tend to practice yoga more, have reported an improved endurance. This is why some athletes will supplement their training with a few sessions of yoga.

Symptom Alleviation and Reduction

Arthritis: If you struggle with arthritis, yoga could be beneficial for your health. According to studies, the slow movement of yoga poses could place gentle pressure on your joints. This deliberate movement could help relieve arthritis symptoms. It is also believed that stress relief could lead to loosening muscles and in return, loosen tight joints.

Cancer: While the research is still being tested, some results showed that cancer patients could benefit greatly from yoga. For those who did practice yoga, some found that they gained strength, and were able to raise the number of red blood cells in their body. The cancer patients also found that they had a better well-being.

Migraines: We've all been there. That terrible pounding in your head that you just can't shake. Try yoga! Some studies have shown that regular yoga practice can lead to a reduced number of migraines for those patients who suffered from chronic migraines.

Constipation: Constipation is something that a majority of people have suffered through at some point in their lives. Did you know that yoga can lead to better posture? Through having a better posture, your digestive and elimination systems will work better. It also helps if you have a healthier diet which normally comes hand in hand when one is exercising.

Obsessive Compulsive Disorder: Some recent studies have shown that for those with OCD that practice yoga, had a reduction in symptoms. For these individuals, fewer symptoms then lead to less medication and even no medication at all.

Back Pain: Do you experience chronic back pain? Yoga can help. Due to some of the positions held in yoga, they can help reduce spinal compression, leading to reduced back pain. Be sure to stick around for later in the chapter when we give you a step-by-step program on how to get started with the basic of yoga.

Body Chemistry Benefits

Vitamin C: A majority of us are aware that it is Vitamin C that can help boost your immunity, but did you also know that the powerful antioxidant also helps produce collagen? Some studies have shown that for those who practice yoga daily, have an increase of Vitamin C in their body, leading to a healthier immune system!

Endocrine: For those who practiced yoga, they found that it helped control their hormone secretion. An improved system allows for your body to keep your hormones in balance, therefore leading to a better physical and emotional health.

Red Blood Cells: We touched on this when we mentioned that yoga could help cancer patients, so here are the facts. Yoga studies have shown that the practice can lead to an increased level of red blood cells. Red blood cells are the reason that oxygen is able to get into the bloodstream. A higher red blood count can lead to better energy!

Triglycerides: Yes, the chemical form of fat. For those who have an elevated triglyceride level, have a higher risk for both heart disease as well as a higher blood pressure. Did you know that yoga can help lower these levels? Yes, indeed!

Lymphatic System: This system is in charge of your immune system. It is supposed to make sure that it gets rid of the toxins in your body. Luckily for yoga people, the movement of yoga gets the system flowing, promoting a very strong lymphatic system.

Emotional Benefits:

Mood: Many of us suffer from mood swings. Our mood can be affected by the smallest of events. Yoga can change this. Those who practice yoga have been known to have a stronger mind and body connection and have the ability to focus inward, therefore granting the ability to improve the mood.

Self-acceptance: As we just mentioned, the focus of yoga is on an inward glance. The point of yoga is not to be perfect, but to accept yourself as you are. Yoga gives you the ability to learn how to love yourself, love your body, and accept your place in the world.

Hostility: People who practice yoga reported a reduction in the hostility they feel when they do become angry. This is because yoga gives a calming effect that leads to relaxation and can calm the nervous system. A calmer nervous system also leads to a lower blood pressure, making a yogi less stressed and have a much healthier approach to life's problems.

Self-Control: A big aspect of yoga is having controlled movements as you go from pose to pose. This idea can be taken out of the yoga room and with you into your daily life. Once you learn self-control from yoga, you can apply it to all aspects of your life.

Positive View of Life: When yoga grants you the ability to become relaxed, happy, and stress-free, it is easy to see why people practicing yoga have such a positive outlook on life. Yoga can balance hormones, giving you a more stable and positive look at life. After all, when you can control your emotions, there is a lot less to get upset over.

Other Health Benefits

Posture: You've learned the benefits for in and out the body, but there is so much more that yoga has to offer. The nature of yoga is meant to promote how to hold one's body. This practice can lead to a better posture, therefore making you look healthier and more confident!

More Energy: Most of you probably feel tired after exercising. With yoga, if it is done correctly, it can lead to feeling more energized after. Negative energy can bring you down and make you feel exhausted. Once you let go of the bad thoughts and relax, you will feel the energy flowing right back to you.

Balance: If you know anything about yoga, it is

you will realize that it takes great balance. As you practice yoga, you may notice an improved balance in and outside of your session. Yoga's main focus is to have control over your body.

Sleep: Do you always find yourself lacking sleep? Do you find your thoughts racing as soon as you lay down? Perhaps you just can't get comfortable? A yoga routine may change your life. Yogi's have found that the practice of yoga can help induce sleep and get you to sleeping better and falling asleep faster.

Sexuality: Yes, you read that correctly. The practice of yoga can help lead to a better sex life! Why you may ask? Through yoga practice, you will be learning better control, a better sense of relaxation, and an improvement in self-confidence. With all of these benefits, they could be divulging onto your partner, leading to a better sex life!

At this point, you're basically like, "I get it! There are amazing benefits of yoga, let's just get started already!" You're finally here. We hope we made our point that yoga can help you not only relax, but also has so many other amazing benefits. The yoga sequence about to follow has a main focus on being mindful with an emphasize on balance. We suggest this sequence for first thing when you wake up, or just before you go to bed. It is gentle, relaxing, and a great way to get started on your yoga journey. We hope to improve your strength, flexibility, as well as your stamina. Now, enjoy our step by step guide to getting you started with beginner's yoga!

FIRST: Remember how we suggested getting started before? We want you to find your happy place. Be sure you find a space that in comfortable and quiet. Once there, set up your mat or your cushion, and let's get started.

Basic Poses

What follows is a set of poses that you can follow as a sequence from the Hand Walking to the Standing pose. We will also have an alternative set of poses that you can follow in the next section.

1. **Hand Walking**

Once you find your spot, sit down on your knees. Please start by focusing on your breath. Breathe in. Breathe out. Feel as the air fills your lungs and then exits through your nostrils. After about five minutes, bring your focus back to your body, back to the room, and you are ready to begin the first position.

Hand walking is very simple. All you are going to be doing is place your right hand on the floor in front of you, followed by your left hand. You will want to walk your hands out one after another until you are in a knee-plank position. Once you are on all fours, you are ready for the next part of the sequence.

2. Finding your Balance

At this point, you should be on all fours like a cat or a dog. Take some time in this position to feel how your weight is distributed. If you feel you have more weight in your hands, shift back a little bit. Your balance should be directly in your core. In this position, go ahead and move around. Practice shifting your weight from your right hand to your right knee. Next, shift your weight from your left hand to your left knee. Feel yourself have complete control over your body. You are the reason it is moving. You have complete control over your being. Remember that.

3. The Cow Pose

On the third pose, you should still be on your hands and knees. You already took control of your body and are aware that you are the one in control. Now, take a deep breath in. Feel how you should be controlling your breath in this new position. As you inhale, lift your seat and your chest. As your chest goes up, feel as your spine drops into your belly and toward the earth. Feel the stretch down your back and enjoy the way your body moves into this position. Stay in this position for a few beats before you move into number four, the Cat Pose.

4. The Cat Pose

Once you come out of the Cow Pose, be sure to let your breath go. Feel as the air exits through your nostrils, giving you life. Now, reverse the curve of your back and lift your waist to the sky. As you do this, be sure to drop your head and your tail to the earth.

Now that you have the Cow and Cat sequence, please repeat this between 5 and 10 times. Take the time to feel your body as it moves through the motions. Notice how your spine curves one way and then the other. You do NOT need to be perfect! You should be moving in a way that makes you comfortable, happy, and relaxed. Once you have moved through this sequence as many times as you want, we move to the next step.

5. Standing Pose

To do the Cow/Cat Pose, simply rerun the first step and walk your hands back, one at a time. Once in sitting position, take some time to concentrate on your breathing. Feel as your spine relaxes in this position. Now, come back into the position on all fours and feel your weight transfer into all fours. Once comfortable, you are ready to stand up.

Remember that yoga is all about the flow of moves, connecting your mind, your body, and your soul. To stand up, step your right hand back, your left hand back, and then shift your weight onto your feet to help you stand up. However, do not stand straight up. Allow yourself to bring your head up gradually, rolling your spine up block by block. Feel the physical sensation of your spine stacking as you stand tall, and then take a deep breath in.

6. Standing Shoulder Rotation

Now that you are standing, it is time to feel your body in this position. To start, you will want to extend your arms out to both of your sides and then roll your palms, so they are face up. Once in position, be sure to exhale and roll your palms back. Feel as your body moves at your will, be grateful for the opportunity to be able to roll your shoulders back and forth. Feel your muscles relax and loosen as you stretch them back and forth.

7. Standing Side Bends

Now, bring your arms back down to your side. Close your eyes as you inhale and exhale, bringing the attention back to your whole body. When you are ready, open your eyes and allow yourself to move into this next position.

To begin, you will want to inhale and bring one arm over your head. As you exhale, bend your body to the right and then inhale as you bring your body back to the neutral position. Inhale again to bring your other arm over your head and then exhale as you bend to the left. You will want to repeat this position several times as you move from side to side. Be sure you are aware of your body as it bends to your will. Remember to only bend as far as you are comfortable. You never need to push yourself, especially as a beginner. The idea is to get comfortable with the movements and relax into them.

8. Standing

You have reached the end of this short beginner's sequence. While you are standing, bring your attention back to your body. Feel as you ground yourself in your environment and focus on your breathing. Feel your breath as it comes in and out of your nostrils. Once you have found your breath, give yourself a pat on the back. You have made it through your first yoga sequence. Eventually, you will be able to make your way through more difficult positions. For now, you are well on your way!

Alternative Basic Poses and Warm-up

This is an alternative Basic set of poses and warm up routine. You can use either this alternate set of poses or the set of poses in the basic set above.

1. Mountain Pose

- Stand straight with your feet together and relax your shoulders. Distribute your weight evenly to both your feet through your soles. Keep your arms at your sides and your fingers together.
- Close your eyes and take a deep breath. Inhale for about five seconds, hold for three seconds and exhale for eight seconds.
- Raise your hands overhead. Stretch your arms up, palms facing each other.
- Slowly lift up your heels and stand on your toes. Inhale and exhale using the same breathing technique, but this time, move your arms and heels down while you exhale.

Tip: For first timers, you may find it a challenge to keep your feet together. If so, don't push yourself too hard. To keep your balance, you can spread your feet. For your next session try to move your feet closer.

2. Downward Dog

- Stand on your hands and knees. Your arms right under your shoulders and knees under your hips. Your back, head, and buttocks should be parallel to the floor.
- Adjust your hands a few inches forward. Keep your fingers apart and press your palms against the mat.
- Inhale, and while exhaling, slowly lift your knees off the floor, pressing your hips toward the ceiling. Next, bring your body into an inverted V and shift your weight to your legs and feet.
- Slightly bend your knees, move your feet apart and move your shoulders away from your ears.
- Take deep breaths. Keep your body in this position as long as you can. Once done, slowly curl your knees and place it back on the floor while you exhale.

Tip: It's ok to shift the weight to your elbows if your arms aren't able to support upper body weight. Just make an attempt slowly. You can use one of your yoga like pillows below your head, so you can rest your forehead while you are in this position.

3. Warrior

- Start by doing a basic mountain pose. As you stand, keep your legs apart and twist your feet to the side.
- Bring your hands to your hips and relax your shoulders. Spread your hands in a straight line by extending your arms sideways with your palm facing down.
- Slowly bend your right knee 90 degrees, lowering your upper body, and align your shoulder to the same direction. Gaze out over your right hand.
- Keep your body in this position for one minute as you take deep breaths.
- Gently move to original pose. Switch sides and repeat.

Tip: On your first few sessions, you may feel a little pain on your knee while you take on this basic pose, that's normal. All you have to do is raise your thighs higher, and since you're just starting, you don't have to keep it parallel it to the floor. It'll get more comfortable over time and through continued practice.

4. Bridge

- Lie down on your back. Bend your knees directly you're your heels.
- Place your arms at your sides with the palms of your hands facing down. Take a deep breath. Exhale and then press feet and arms on the floor as you push your hips upward. Raise your rear as high as possible.
- Hold this position for at least a minute. Slowly Exhale and gently bring your body back to the floor or mat.

  Tip: To make this pose easier to perform, place a pillow on your back, underneath your tailbone. Do not try and force your thighs parallel to the floor. If it's a challenge for you, then take your time, you can always try it another day.

5. Triangle

- Assume the basic mountain pose. Extend your arms to your sides, and bend over your right leg.
- Stand with feet apart, turn your right foot's toes to 90 degrees, and your left foot to 45 degrees. Take a deep breath. Lean your body to the right as you exhale.
- Allow your right hand to touch your ankle. Raise your left hand up, extending your fingertips to the

ceiling. Gaze at your fingers that are suspended in the air.

- Keep your body in this position for at least twenty seconds while you take five deep breaths. Slowly transition to the warrior pose as you exhale.
- Stand and repeat on left side.

Tip: If you're unable to reach your ankle, it's ok. Try to reach or touch the shin or calf of your leg instead. Or, you can opt to use straps, tie it around your ankles and reach for it. Gazing up at your fingers can make you feel dizzy at times, but you can close your eyes or stare down to make you feel better.

6. Chair Pose

- Assume the basic mountain pose. Keep your feet together, with your big toes touching. Inhale and lift your arms above your head. Exhale as you bend your knees and body to a 45-degree angle.
- While bending your knee, push your butt and hips lower. Stretch your arms as far as you can. Shift your weight into your heels. This would allow you to lift your toes off the mat if you wanted to.
- Bring your butt lower and hold position up to one minute. For a deeper pose, tilt your head slightly and gaze at a point between your hands.

- Take deep breaths. As you exhale, return to mountain pose.

   Tip: Placing a chair at your back while doing this routine can help you in this pose. This can serve as your guide on how deep you should push your rear down.

7. Seated Twist

- Extend your legs as you sit on the floor or mat. Crossover your right leg to the left and place your right foot outside the left thighs and bend the knee. Your right knee should always point toward the ceiling.
- Keep your back straight. Inhale, and as you exhale, put your left elbow on the outside of your right knee and your right hand on the floor behind you.
- Take deep breaths, twist right and reach your back as far as you can. Make sure to keep both sides of your rear on the floor.
- Inhale, take a deep breath and hold the position as long as you can. Untwist your back as you exhale. Switch sides and repeat.

   Tip: At all times, keep your bottom leg straight and place both hands on your raised knee. You can tuck your feet near your rear if you find it uncomfortable to sit on your feet. While you twist your body, do it slowly and do not outstretch your back.

8. Cobra Pose

- Lie down on your stomach, with the chin on the floor. Place your palms flat on the floor under your shoulders and legs.
- Press your pubic bone down as you lift your head and shoulders. Kee your hips down as you squeeze your glutes. Keep your shoulders down and loose. Don't tense or squeeze your shoulders up to your ears.
- Use your hands to help arch your head and chest as high as you can.
- Breathe and hold the position for 2 to 6 breaths.
- As you exhale, bring your chest and head lower to the floor. Relax and repeat procedure.

  Tip: Always move within a pain-free range of motion and with control. Do not push yourself too hard especially in lifting your upper body higher. Take it slow and attempt to lift higher in the next sessions.

9. Child's Pose

- Assume a kneeling position. Sit comfortably on your heels.

- Inhale and Roll your torso forward, bringing your forehead to rest on the floor or mat. Lower your body towards your knees as you exhale.
- Slowly extend your arms in front of you and reach as far as possible. Close your eyes. Breathe and hold the position for 2 to 3 minutes.
- Shift your hands back to your sides. Reach back as far as you can. Stay in this position until you feel relaxed.
- Gently raise your body and go back to a kneeling position.

Tip: As an extension of the floor, you can use a pillow if you're not flexible enough to have your head rest on the floor. If your abs are making it a little uneasy for you to assume this position, then raise your rear a little higher instead so that your head can touch the floor.

Warm-up Routines for Yoga

You must be pretty excited after determining the basic poses of Yoga and how to do it properly. Still, we have a lot more to discuss, especially warm-up routines.

Just like in any other exercises, warm-ups are very important. It serves as a preparation to make you and your body ready for an activity. Disregarding warm-ups can cause injured tissues and health problems. To keep your going, here are some warm-up routines you can do before Yoga. Don't worry; it's simple.

Eye Exercise

- Look up and down; right and left counting to 8 for each position.
- Look in the upper left and upper right; lower left and lower right, counting to   8 for each position.
- Roll your eyes clockwise four times and do the same counterclockwise.
- Repeat the routine twice.

Face Exercise

- First, expand your cheeks by filling your mouth with air. Slowly release the air from your mouth after taking four deep breaths.
- Suck your cheek in as much as you can. Then take four deep breaths and slowly release your cheek.
- Open your mouth and smile widely. Using your fingers, pull the skin on the edge of your lips up and take four deep breaths. Remove your finger on the edge of your lips and pull the lips into a

point. Pull as far as possible. Slowly return your lips to a normal shape after taking four deep breaths.

- Open your mouth as wide as you can. As your mouth opens, raise your eyebrows and take four deep breaths. Form an "o" with your lips as you breathe four times. Now, while hiding your teeth, try to smile. Again, breathe four times and then relax your lips.

- Pull your head back and stretch out your neck. While doing so, you should push your chin as far as you can. Take four deep breaths and pull your chin in. After taking four breaths, rest your chin.

Neck Exercise

- To Start with, pull your head back as far as you can. After that, pull it down to your chest until your chin touches your chest. Breathe four times and as you straighten you head, exhale.

- Move and twist your head from left to right on eight counts in each position.

- Rotate your neck clockwise and counterclockwise; repeat three times.

Shoulder and Hand Exercise

- Raise your shoulders as high as you can. Stay in this position as you take four breaths. Now, lower your shoulders to rest on your last exhale.
- Pull your shoulders far back and tightly squeeze your shoulder blades. Then, take four breaths and rest your shoulders as you exhale.
- Rotate your shoulders forward and backward doing eight counts in each direction.
- Using a yoga strap, hold its edges and measure the width of your shoulder. Place it above your legs and lift your arms up to your chest. Pull your hands back up as far as you can at the same time you inhale. Return your arms to your chest while you exhale and repeat the procedure four or five times.
- Join your fingertips without your palms touching and spread it as wide as you can. Push it outwards and extend your hands far out. Repeat eight times.

Knee and Feet Exercise

- Sit on a chair and make yourself comfortable. Raise your right foot and move it from side to side on eight times. Rest your right foot and do the same routine with your left foot. Repeat three or four times.

- Still sitting on a chair, raise your right foot and rotate your ankle clockwise eight times. Rest your foot and do the same routine on your left foot. Repeat three or four times.

Breathing Exercise

- Assume a cross-sitting position. Place your right hand above your chest and your left hand on your stomach (or visa verse).
- Count to five as you breathe in deeply. When you inhale, use your hand to push your stomach in and hold your breath for three seconds.
- Exhale slowly up to the count of eight. While doing this, slightly push your chest in using your hand and relax the other hand on your stomach. Repeat this routine at least five times.

Note: Before jumping right into yoga poses or routine, make sure to do this first. It's a must. Once you're done doing this for about 10-15 minutes, you are now ready to take on proper yoga routines.

Basic Routines That Work Best

Basic Yoga routines utilize the most basic poses that we have discussed previously. It may also include some poses that weren't mentioned above, but we will tackle it along the way. There are three basic routines: standing, sitting and lying. We'll discuss it one by one.

- **Basic Standing Routine**

1.   Assume mountain pose. Raise your arms and hold your position for 15 seconds.

2.   Assume prayer pose by lowering your hands slowly to your chest. breath in and then slowly lift your praying hands above your head again and breath out. At the same time, place your left foot on your right thigh. Hold your pose for a minute.

3.   Slowly, lower your hands and your thighs. Then, assume prayer pose again.

4.   Using your right foot and left thigh, follow step #2 and step #3 again.

5.   From the prayer pose, slowly transition to basic warrior pose by sliding your left foot to the back. Extend your hands at shoulder level and perform 6-8 twists.

6.   Next, return to prayer pose. Then, redo step #5, this time, use your right foot.

7.   After your last twist, assume basic triangle pose. Hold this pose for each side for 15-20 seconds.

8.   Slowly return to prayer pose and transition to mountain pose.

9.   Assume the forward bend pose. (Stand with your feet together and bend your knees slightly and bend your body from the waist forward. Place your hands or fingertips on your toes.

- **Basic Sitting Routine**

1. From the forward bend pose, slowly take on the squat pose by lowering your rear.

2. Now transition to an easy pose (seated position with your rear on the floor, then do a simple cross-legged sitting position, placing the feet directly below the knees). Perform 5 breathing exercise while assuming this pose.

3. From the easy pose, do the half-twist pose. Hold this pose for each leg for 15-20 seconds. Perform two sets of the half-twist pose.

4. Stretch your legs together and do the forward bend pose while sitting. As you bend, don't forget to exhale.

5. Gently raise your torso and do the seated twist pose. Stay in this position for 15-20 seconds and perform two sets of this routine.

6. Using your arms as support, curl your knees a little. Slowly lie on the floor or mat and continue with the basic corpse pose (This is dead simple, you lie down on your back and relax your body and mind).

- **Basic Lying Routine**

1. Continue doing the corpse pose, then raise your left leg perpendicularly to your body. Breathe and hold your position for 15 to 20 seconds. Now, with your right leg, redo the procedure.

2. Go back to the corpse pose smoothly.

3. This time, raise both of your legs together and stay in this position for 10 to 15 seconds. While your legs are still suspended in the air, make the scissors motion eight times. After that, continue raising your legs together.

4. Gently pull your knees towards your chest. Perform the gas release pose (press your curled knees tightly to your chest, and you wrap your hands around your shin).

5. Slowly, free your legs and transition back to corpse pose.

6. Curl your legs one more time and proceed to the basic bridge position. Perform this pose for 15-20 seconds and redo it three times.

7.   Once completed, return to the basic corpse pose and place your hand behind under your rear. Lift your chest calmly while pulling your head back as far as possible (Fish pose). Stay in this position for 15-20 seconds and repeat three times.

8.   Return to the basic corpse pose. Rest for a minute or two and take deep breaths. Turn to your side and slowly assume a sitting position. Then transition to the basic mountain pose.

You have successfully completed the routine.

Note: These are just basic routines that you can do. It will also work well for weight loss. For advanced routines, you can go ahead and research about Sun and Moon Salutations. This routine has numerous healing and health benefits.

Other Yoga Poses for Relaxation

If you do not have the time to sit down for a yoga sequence, try practicing some of these other moves to get a calm mind!

Upavistha Konasana- Seated Wide Angle Pose

For this position, you will want to be sitting on the floor, a couch, or even your bed. You can begin by having your legs spread wide apart while having a pillow placed in front of your torso. As you sit up, begin to inhale so that you are as tall as possible. As you exhale, please fold your body forward until it is resting on the pillow in front of you. If you cannot reach forward, feel free to place a soft bend in your knees. Stay in this position as you breathe in and out about ten times. Once you feel relaxed, take a deep breath as you inhale and rise back up to the seated position.

Supta Baddha Konadana- Reclined Bound Angle Pose

While sitting on your bed, take a position on your back with a pillow lengthwise beneath you. Once you are comfortable, try bringing the soles of your feet together and allow for your knees to drop to the side. As you exhale, recline your body toward the earth and allow yourself to sink as you stretch your inner hip. Stay here for about two minutes or until you are ready to sit up on your own. Be sure to concentrate on your breathing and feel connected to the earth.

Jathara Parivartanasana- Supine Spinal Twist

For this movement, you should be in the

same position as the reclined bound angle pose. Be sure that your back is supported by the pillow before moving into Jathara Parivartanasana. Once in position, gently drop both of your knees to the side while using your hands. Be sure to have your arms by your side with palms facing up. From this point, allow for your breath to act like a wave coming over your spine. With each exhale, you will want to release the tension from your body. We invite you to stay in this position for a few minutes before coming to a neutral stance, followed by dropping the knees to the other side. Remember that for most of these positions, what you do on one side, you will want to do to the other.

Viparite Karani- Legs Up The Wall

For the viparite karani, you will want to set a pillow against the wall before you lay down on top of it. Be sure that your seat bones are directed at the wall before you extend your legs up toward the ceiling. Now, keep your feet stacked over your hips and allow for your head and shoulder to rest on either the floor or your mattress. Once in position, try extending your arms by your side while having your palms facing the sky. This position will feel especially grand if you spend a lot of time on your feet. Your legs up on the wall can create a healing effect on your body while improving the circulation. We invite you to stay in this position for 2-3 minutes before bending your knees, rolling to one side, and finally sitting up.

<u>Savasana- Corpse Pose</u>

We suggest this pose a last pose in your yoga routine. Whether you are looking to relax before bed, or still need to move on through your day, be sure to take advantage of this peaceful moment while you breathe and settle back into your body. Simply lay down while extending your legs in front of you. Once lying down, please take your left hand and place it over your heart, while taking your right hand and placing it over your stomach. Now, take the time to breathe deep and come back to your place in the world. You should feel relaxed and ready to face what tackle anything that may come your way!

Do's and Don'ts To Follow For An Injury-Free Routine

Yoga is much like any other activities; it also has its rules or do's and don'ts that should be followed at all times. It is a gentle routine, but it requires delicacy to avoid injuries or any harm to the body. "better safe than sorry." Being aware of things around you can really save your life. Here are significant guidelines you ought to know.

Do's:

- The best times to practice yoga are: early in the morning, after taking a shower and without eating anything.
- You can perform yoga before a shower, however, after practice, you must rest first. Wait for a while and then take a shower.
- Let fresh air in the room and light fill the room while performing yoga.
- When practicing yoga, face east or north in the morning, west or south in the evening. Always remember to spread and sit on a yoga mat, a blanket, a carpet, or a clean cloth.
- While doing yoga, you must concentrate only on yoga and try to keep away from unwanted thoughts.
- You should practice yoga calmly. Haste or exhaustion defeats the purpose of yoga. If you feel tired, you should rest in a comfortable posture.
- Always lay on your back after finishing poses for 2 to 5 minutes with relaxed breathing.

- Wipe your sweat off either by using a cloth or with your palms to avoid slipping on it if it sticks to the floor.

Don'ts:

- Sudden movements should be avoided during Yoga sessions. You have to move slowly especially when shifting poses.
- Don't perform Yoga right after eating. Wait a couple of hours; then you can do your Yoga routine.
- Don't take a shower or drink water for 30 minutes after doing yoga.
- If suffering from any illness, sprain or fracture, you should refrain from Yoga practice and always ask for professional medical when it is safe to return to practicing Yoga.
- Do not resist help from an instructor or someone who has more knowledge than you. This will do a great deal in preventing injury and avoiding getting hurt especially when working on routines and poses.
- Don't bring your cellphones or tablets inside the studio. You have to leave socializing and business outside the studio, so the peace of the practice is not disturbed. Plus, it will cause a distraction, and you might end up losing your balance.

- Don't push yourself too hard. If you can't perform as deeply or completely into a pose as others might be able to do, don't you ever force yourself to your limits to avoid straining or injuring yourself.
- Don't wear excessive garments for your routine. Just wear comfortable clothes that would allow you to move freely.

Chapter Four: Mindfulness-based Cognitive Therapy (MBCT)

As we mentioned earlier, there is this program known as Mindfulness-based Cognitive Therapy. So, what is it exactly?   It was first designed to prevent a patient from relapsing into depression. MBCT was specifically made for those who suffered from major depressive disorder (MDD). Mindfulness-based Cognitive Therapy was created specifically for this disorder whereas mindfulness-based stress reduction is applied to a broader range of disorders as we will be covering later in this chapter.

MBCT uses a lot of the traditional cognitive behavioral therapy methods while adding newer strategies including mindfulness meditation as you learned about in an earlier chapter. While the cognitive methods educate the patient about depression, what it is, and how it is affecting their chemical balance and body, mindfulness meditation focuses on becoming aware of these thoughts and feelings. As you learned earlier, the point of being mindful is to accept the feelings. However, rather than accepting them for what they are, the patient must learn to neither attach themselves or react to these feelings. This whole process is known as 'decentering." After the session, the patient learns that they must disengage themselves from the moods and rumination that comes from negative thinking.

The whole concept behind MBCT is to learn how to pay attention to your feelings and then concentrate on everything with a purpose. A patient must remember that each moment that they are alive is important and that they cannot judge themselves off of one situation or one feeling. By being mindful, a patient can understand that while being depressed, holding onto the negative feelings is both ineffective and can be mentally destructive.

The program itself was developed to target depressive relapse for a number of reasons. First, the MBCT program can help a patient learn how to manage their mind and gain skills toward metacognitive awareness. In doing so, they can accept their negative thought pattern and try to respond in a more skillful way. During their sessions, the depression patients decenter their thoughts through a different pattern so that they can become conscious of their emotional process.

The MBCT program lasts about eight weeks and is a group intervention. During these two months, the patients take a two hour weekly courses and then after the fifth week, they attend a day long class. The point of the classes is to have the patients practice what they learn outside of their class. By using guided meditation, they can add mindfulness into their daily lives.

We had also mentioned Mindfulness-based stress reduction earlier or MBSR. This is a mindfulness-based program which was designed to help people with a range of conditions, pain, and life issues. The program has a combination of body awareness, mindfulness meditation, as well as yoga. In this part of the book, you are an expert on both of these! As you already know, yoga and meditation both have the beneficial effects of improved quality of life, relaxation, and great stress reduction. However, though we know that there isn't solid evidence that the program can prevent or cure any diseases, studies have shown that it can help despite the spiritual roots of MBSR.

The whole program was designed by Kabat-Zinn, who stated that the point of mindfulness is to live "moment-to-moment, nonjudgmental awareness." This is why during the program, the patients have to focus on incorporating the mindfulness activities into their daily routines. By doing so, they were able to heighten their sensitivity to not only their environment but also to their reaction to it. By becoming aware, the patients were able to enhance their coping skills along with their self-management skills. It was the therapy that allowed them to escape their feelings of the past and worry about the future.

Similar to MBCT, the program is an eight-week session where there are weekly group meetings with two-hour classes followed by a one-day retreat. However, they have 45 minutes of homework where they are asked to practice three formal techniques. These include simple yoga moves, body scanning, and mindfulness meditation. Body scanning is a new term for us and is one of the first techniques taught at this workshop. All it is is lying on your back while focusing your attention on a certain body part. Most times, this will start at the toes and then move the focus up to the top of your head. This practices the control over your mind and your body, giving you the connection for both.

Chapter Five: Tips on Mindfulness for Beginners

1. **Prioritize being Mindful**
   Just like anything in life, you may not get very far if you don't make mindfulness an important aspect of your life.

2. **Slow Down**
   Many of us move through our lives quickly. We are taught to be as productive as possible and to always multi-task when you can. Mentally, this can be exhausting. In today's society obsessed with speed, take the time to slow down. Instead of rushing around, realize that there are other ways to live your life. Life doesn't have to be fast-paced, passing you by. Be mindful of your time and take some time to meditate. Look at how beautiful life is and how lucky we are to be alive right now.

3. **Take Time to Sit**
   As we mentioned earlier, many of us rush through our lives. We invite you to take the time to sit down during your morning, your lunch break, or any free moment you get. Adopting some daily practice into your schedule is very important. You

can take the time to sit in a quiet zone and be free of distractions to reset yourself. Remember, the more practice you get, the easier it will become.

4. Be Easy

With that being said, remember that while being mindful, you need to become nonjudgmental, especially of yourself. The concept is about an acceptance of everything. Accept the thoughts, sensations, and feelings that may be in your mind. Remember that they are neither good nor bad. When you are mindful, you are just an observer of your emotions and thoughts. You should not get flustered if you cannot hold your concentration just yet. The world is full of distractions. Keep practicing, and you will become more in control of your body as time goes on.

5. Patience is a Virtue

You are not going to be an expert on mindfulness, meditation, or yoga in just a couple of day, weeks or even months. You need to practice. It takes both time and patience to develop your skills. When you first start, you may feel a little more present and a little more alive, but also expect to feel flustered. With more practice, you will have these feelings and the ability to grow. The more you work on it, the stronger it will get, just like your muscles. In time, and you will have peace and happiness in your life.

6. Develop your Concentration

To practice mindfulness, remember that concentration is a lot like an anchor. It is the point which keeps you together in the moment. It is the active force that can have you focus on your breath, your environment, and your body. Try thinking of mindfulness as your field of vision. At first, you should place your concentration on your breathing and then to your body. As you exercise your concentration abilities, mindfulness will become easier for you. To start, just concentrate on your breath. This can be done just about anywhere. Whether you are at a stop light, cleaning dishes, or sitting for your meditation session. Concentrate on your breath and build your endurance to enhance your mindfulness skills.

7. Remember to Have Fun

While you may be busy trying to get better at mindfulness, meditation, and yoga, remember to have fun! Luckily for us, it normally comes naturally while we are learning. Not only are you bettering yourself, but you are also learning a new skill. Once you have got it down, you may feel a sense of utter tranquility. Gaining a sense of peace in this mad world is not something everyone can accomplish! Just remember that in the beginning, you will have to push yourself to finish each session.

8. Let it Go

NO, we don't mean that you have to belt at the top of your lungs while you run away to your magical ice castle. When you first get started with mindful meditation, we can promise that it will be difficult. We have been mentioning this time and time again through this whole book. Remember, it is going to happen. You are going to get distracted. Let It Go! There is nothing in life that we are instantly good at. The point is to be mindful of these distractions, accept them, and then let them go. The more you practice, the easier it will be to let these thoughts and feelings go. Eventually, you will lose the frustration and move on with peace, dignity, and relaxation.

9. Keep it Simple

As a beginner you would want, to begin with, the basics and then move on from there. This is why we are going to suggest mindful breathing for the first few weeks. Breathing is easy; you've been doing it since day one! Now, all you need to do is be mindful of your breath. As you move on, remember that breathing is the base of mindfulness meditation. Try taking 10 to 15 minutes in your morning and before bed to practice breathing. Eventually, you will be able to move to other practices such as mindful walking and mindful eating. The main idea is that you do not need to rush to develop a mindful life. Start basic and work your way up. You will be happy you did!

Chapter 6: Yoga Diet

A good and healthy diet with help fulfill your yoga practice. You have to support your body through healthy eating. It is part of the Yogi belief that food is the creator of Prana, a life force that nurtures our bodies and provides us vitality and good health. This is why the food that we eat plays a crucial role in increasing prana and a higher state of consciousness. Some experts assert that to maximize your mind and body's full potential. You should consume a yogic diet with proper physical posture (asana), breathing techniques (pranayama) and meditation.

You might be surprised that a lot of food which you like, is included in the list of sustenance that should be avoided to follow a strict yoga diet. Check out ten foods that you should start taking off your list according to Lisa Mitchell, of MindBodyGreen.

- Meat, fish, and eggs
- junk food, Processed food,
- soda, candy, and other high sugar content foods.
- artificial sweeteners,
- margarine
- White flour
- Fried food
- Garlic, onions, spicy foods
- Burnt, moldy or rotting food
- Microwaved foods
- Alcohol, tobacco, stimulants

You might be a little shocked and bewildered right now. However, if you really are determined to pursue Yoga, this is a part of the discipline that you have to instill within yourself. Nobody said that you should get rid of these foods from your system right away. You can start by avoiding one food at a time and eventually, you'll master this diet.

Furthermore, foods are classified into three different types, according to Yogic diet, namely:

- Sattvic food is food which purifies the body and calms the mind, like green leafy vegetables, fresh fruits, nuts, grains, fresh milk, certain spices. Aside from that, cooked food that is consumed within 3-4 hours can also be classified under this category.
- Rajasic food - stimulates the body and mind into action but if taken in excess, it can be bad. It can cause hyperactivity, restlessness, anger, irritability, and sleeplessness. Spicy food, onion, garlic, tea, coffee, fried food is considered to be Rajasic foods.
- Tamasic food – this type of food can cause dullness of the mind which may result in inertia, confusion, and disorientation. Foods under this classification are mostly oily or heavy food and food containing artificial preservatives.

Of course, sattvic foods are the highly recommended ones. Also, a Yogic diet requires the right kind of food that brings about light feeling and makes you feel energetic. This diet plan requires plenty of salads, fresh vegetables, fresh fruits, milk and raw nuts. Include these items in your existing dietary choices. Plus, you must avoid overeating or the intake of unnecessary food in between meals.

Once again, you don't have to be a vegan to practice Yoga. It only says to avoid or reduce eating meat or poultry products, which means that you can still eat meat once in a while. Following the Yogic diet and incorporating it into Yoga practice can put your health at its maximum level.

Tip: Eat slowly and chew your food thoroughly so that you can make your food more digestible. This will also allow the nutrients and healthy components of the food to be easily absorbed by our body.

The Pathway to A Healthier Life

Nowadays, more and more people are spending for a better way of life, especially in health. Some even spend thousands of dollars just to ensure that their health is not compromised given their chosen lifestyle. Not everyone can spend that much money to secure well-being, though. Aside from expensive medical solutions or procedures, there are a number of ways to achieve your goals, such as doing physical activities or exercises. Some may say that you have to go to the gym and sweat it out to get fit or reduce risks of getting diseases and promote good health. However, this statement is not completely true. Most of the best exercises that can do wonders to your wellness don't require the gym. To name a few are swimming, walking or other aerobic exercises, Tai Chi an example of balance exercise, and lastly Yoga.

Yoga is considered as a flexibility exercise, which provides you more freedom of movement for other exercises and for your everyday activities. According to research, it is one of the best ways to lose weight and get fit, and it is far better than gym workouts, and it is way cheaper. It is also good for pregnant women, given the right poses. According to Harvard Health Publications, the total number of calories you can burn in this exercise depends on your body weight. So for example, if you weigh 125 pounds, at the end of a

Mindfulness With Yoga

30-minute yoga session you'll burn 120 calories, and if you weigh 185 pounds, it will be 178 calories.

One of the major advantages of Yoga is improved overall health. We have mentioned a number of times that Yoga is more than just an exercise, and leading a healthier life is just one of the few it could offer you, in the best way you could ever imagine. It has the potential to be the single most effective form of physical fitness there is.

Yes, you can opt to do Yoga at home (which I know is more convenient for you), however, it is still safer to attend Yoga classes in a studio, especially if you're a beginner or newbie. Even long time yogis still prefer to do Yoga along with others in studios. This way, you will learn the correct way of executing those poses on routines plus they can assist you in every session on how to improve your posture and movements.

Now, aside from Yoga, good nutrition is an important part of leading a healthy lifestyle. You should be careful of what you put inside your stomach. There will be numerous temptation around you, yet you still have to keep those temptations at bay. I mean, who wouldn't want to grab a bite of those burgers from famous fast food chains? Or a taste of the sumptuous steak meals? It's really hard to resist these mouth-watering foods. However, not all delicious and flavorful snacks are good. Checking the nutritional value of the food you eat is a must. Yes, you can still eat that food but only a little. It's better to avoid them to follow the right path into the life you want.

Additional preservatives found in processed food can contain ingredients that contain toxins and free radicals that can harm your liver and other internal organs. You have to watch what you eat. The fresher the food, the better. When you buy fruits or vegetables, it is best to purchase organic because of the freshness, and it's safe from pesticides.

Valuing health has never been imperative and knowing that in this generation, more diseases and illnesses are surfacing. It is for this particular reason that we all have to change our lifestyle and exercise more. We are no longer getting any younger, so, better start now. Being healthy and enthusiastic to have fun and explore life sounds much better than battling off cancer, obesity, or lifestyle-preventable diseases.

The road to total fitness or healthier life may not be as easy as it sounds. You have to possess a great amount of determination, dedication, and discipline. The moment you decide to take its course, make sure that you're brave enough not to quit on what you have started.

Health is Wealth: Here's What You Can Gain From Yoga

Even as kids, we were taught that "Health is Wealth." This means that being healthy is more important than being rich and sick. When you're healthy, you can do more, and when you are at work, you can accomplish your tasks with high energy. Health is the best investment you'll ever have. If all you think about is work and how to earn money, then you're not making a wise decision. Being able to work and save is a good choice, but you have to think about your wellness as well.

Let's say you work very hard; you have made a significant amount of money. What happens if you fail to prioritize your health and end up being sick? Or suffer from a severe ailment in the long run? Your hard earned money will just be spent on your medication and medical procedures to cure whatever sickens you. Medicines and maintenance supplements will cost much as well. On the other hand, if you embody a healthy lifestyle and exercise, certainly the money that you have saved can be allotted to things that you may have always wanted, and you can enjoy every penny that you have gained. It is something to think about. Many young working professionals find it very difficult in practice.

You don't have to do a lot of workouts to have a good health. Yoga is more than enough. It is equivalent to three different exercises combined, so it can be just what you are looking for. In business or banking, if you invest in something you will earn or gain something in return; the same goes with Yoga. Your investment in this activity will allow you to gain more. Here are the five major things that you can gain with Yoga.

Better B's Are Beneficial For You (Blood Sugar, Blood Pressure, Balance, Bone Health)

Blood Sugar

Mindfulness With Yoga

According to the World Health Organization, diabetes is the 7th leading cause of death in the world. However, significant studies about diabetes show that Yoga can help reduce blood sugar, hence, lessen the risk of diabetes. Yoga is one such ancient measure that can be used to control your blood sugar levels effectively. It can help prevent diabetes and stabilize blood sugar level in diabetic patients.

Regular Yoga exercise can keep your weight in check, can slow the rate of succession of diseases and at the same time reduce the severity of symptoms.

Research also suggests that stress is one of the major reasons for diabetes. Increased levels of stress hormones in studies have been shown to raise blood glucose levels, promote overeating which leads to fat accumulation, then high insulin resistance. However, the practice of Yoga contributes to stress reduction and may moderate the impact of diabetes and improve the action of insulin.

Eastern medicine philosophy suggests that certain yoga poses can help stimulate and massage internal organs, including the pancreas, which produces insulin. It also shows significant results in normalizing endocrine gland function and digestion. A number of researches have been conducted all over the world for years, new and advanced clinical studies provide more evidence that supports the claim of the benefits of Yoga in reducing blood sugar and the risk of diabetes.

Blood Pressure

In as much as Yoga reduces and stabilizes blood sugar, it does the same thing to blood pressure. According to some research studies, 90 to 95% of all cases of high blood pressure are characterized as essential hypertension. This is an independent condition which means that it is not affected by any other ailment conditions. Given this, high blood pressure, for the most part, is preventable.

The most underlying factor that triggers high blood pressure is lifestyle factors under your control. Changes in lifestyle can really help lessen the risk of this disease. Recent studies indicate that keeping your muscles flexible and pliant through regular yoga stretches, may also help keep the arteries pliable and thereby lower blood pressure naturally. Aside from that, an evidence-based integrative research of the Medical Center of Georgia reveals that Yoga offers an effective method of treating hypertension that is non-pharmacologic which can be extremely advantageous and healthy for an individual. Drugs can have serious or dangerous side effects and thus an alternative like Yoga could be a good choice.

Studies have found that yoga can be a very efficient and non-invasive way of reducing high blood pressure for both men and women. It is particularly useful in reducing the diastolic number (the most important number). It suggests that people suffering from high blood pressure should only execute certain poses that are suitable for them and should avoid more complex poses.

Balance

The literal meaning of balance, is more than just standing on one foot. Balance means the prevention of future injuries, improved focus, and relief from stress. Balance poses will also improve balance, both in the body and in the mind. One will also see improves coordination, increases strength and better stability.

Older people tend to lose balance which may result in injuries from falling. However, the practice of Yoga significantly improves our state of balance by strengthening different muscles and joints of the body. Certain balance poses such as arm balances strengthen the wrists, arm and shoulder muscles while standing balance poses fortify the legs and knee joints.

Studies also show that Yoga helps in relieving stress, reducing tension and fatigue, which are the common factors that trigger other diseases. Improved balance in both mind and body allows you to do more, move with ease and lessen the safety threats especially that most of our daily activities require balance. The practice of balance can require a lot of effort; that is why it is a vital part of Yoga, as good balance can protect us against daily falls and mishaps.

Bone Health

Our bones are an essential part of our body. It supports our body and operates in many ways like storing calcium, holding muscles, protect organs, and frames our body. As we age, our bones are most likely to lose density, and it grows weak which makes it difficult to move, unlike when we were younger.

According to research, Yoga poses can help strengthen the bones and build bone strength. It can also help avoid bone diseases like Osteoporosis, and if you already have this condition, it could reduce your abnormality. Research shows, yoga, prevents and in some cases even reverse the process of bone loss.

Expert suggests that low-impact weight-bearing yoga poses promote bone growth to build stronger bones. Poses like the standing pose can build strength in your hips, an area commonly affected by osteoporosis. This also shows significant results in reducing back and neck pains. Before doing so, make sure to consult an expert or ask professional advice to determine the poses that may or may not work for you.

Furthermore, clinical studies reveal that therapeutic Yoga can also help provide simple, gentle movements that gradually develop strength, flexibility, and balance – elements that may be especially beneficial for people with arthritis.

Enjoy The Bounty Of A Deep and Sound Sleep

A deep and sound sleep is harder to achieve nowadays especially with all that's happening in our lives, including stress – and that's not good. Sleep deprivation can lead to higher risk of chronic health problems like high blood pressure, heart disease, and stroke. This is why it is important that we should have good quality sleep.

There are other ways to improve our quality of sleep: reducing caffeine intake, avoiding cigarette smoking, refraining from food consumption 3 to 4 hours before sleep and a lot more. One of the best ways to achieve improved sleep quality is through Yoga, according to research.

Certain poses affect the nervous system and adjust the hormones in our brain which can then lead to a normal sleep cycle. Doing Yoga exercises and routines improve blood circulation throughout the body, nourishing all your organs, tissues and nerves. Researchers found out that Yoga is essential in helping those who suffer chronic insomnia and alleviate other sleeping disorders.

Yoga breathing exercises promote cleansing and nourishment throughout our mind and body, by increased supply of oxygen to every cell in the mind and body. Correspondingly, every nerve strength and fiber of the body and mind get oxygenated, hence relaxed. After a while, relaxation induces good sleep and helps cure insomnia resulting from stress syndromes and other psychosomatic disorders.

Aside from the physical aspect, Yoga exercises also help calm the mind through meditation. Meditation frees the mind from any negativity or toxic substance found in everyday life. It induces deep relaxation up to the core levels of our mind and body. It grants you the liberty to drift from your current disturbed state into a rejuvenated being. A relaxed and calm mind can lead to a good and sound sleep.

Boost The Immune System and Helps You Get Rid Of Common Illnesses

Our body's immune system acts as our

defense system which is composed of countless biological structures and processes that protect us from disease-causing organisms. It is like a fortress that fortifies the body from bacteria and viruses. So, imagine if our immune system is weak, as a result, your body will be prone to ailments. That is why it is imperative that we keep our immune system strong at all times.

Healthy eating habits and proper hygiene are two of the most common factors that can help our body fight against common sickness. Nowadays, food supplements and vitamins offer aid in strengthening our body's immune system. However, we should also accredit other ways to boost our immune system, and Yoga is one of the few. This ancient practice can also help us combat infections strengthening our body's functions and systems.

According to clinical studies, Yoga can help regulate the thyroid and blood pressure levels of men and women, while strengthening the digestive system and easing a woman's menstrual cramps and premenstrual syndrome (PMS). It also improves general all round wellbeing. Certain poses such as backbends and bridge, reinforces the upper spine, thus, activating the thymus gland that rests behind the breastbone and the primary organ for immune function.

It is also the key to making our respiratory system strong enough to fight infections. Breathing exercises and posture help improve the lungs' mechanical efficiency by conditioning the repertory tract that increases the elasticity and strength of the whole lung.

Flexibility and Proper Posture

Do you slouch a lot especially at work? You are not alone. Though it may seem normal, it's not good for your health. Poor body structure may lead to worse conditions such as improper digestion, increases stress levels and back pain. As early as possible, it's best to improve proper posture and increase your body's flexibility to avoid such things from happening.

Regular yoga practice stretches and tones the body muscles and also makes them strong. It's also great for improving your body posture when you stand, sit, sleep or walk. The purpose behind every yoga pose is to stimulate the muscles around the spine. Our spinal cord's main function is to send and receive messages from the brain which triggers the rest of our body, controlling our movement and organ function, it is considered to be the core from which our body operates. As a result of holistic strength building, flexibility also increases as well as improved alignment, the health of your entire body will benefit.

Recent studies revealed that yoga increases flexibility and strength, and also offers relaxation and stress management. Once you have maintained proper posture, the advantages are: it naturally enables you to breathe properly, it encourages good digestion, and it is effective in avoiding mood swings and body pain.

Helps Fight Stress

Stress is caused by several things, such as job deadlines, emotional problems, traffic and people questioning you. Stress is one of the major factors that can trigger other diseases, so if stress levels are reduced then, you may be able to the prevent serious medical issues before they occur.

Research shows that certain exercises like yoga can help control agitation and manage stress, and it can also boost your mood and overall sense of well-being. People who practice yoga frequently states that it helps them to get better sleep, and they feel less stressed. Yoga poses do not only work physical wonders; its routines emphasize on the harmony of mind and body which helps you concentrate and connect with your spirit. That connection will then encourage you to live in the moment and disconnect from the thoughts or things that cause your stress.

Yoga breathing exercises, allows us to fall into what they call the "rest and digest" form, allowing our body and mind the much-needed relief that it needs. Learning to concentrate simply on the sound of your breath as you inhale and exhale evenly and smoothly will help you gently but effectively switch your attention from feelings of anxiety to feelings of relaxation.

Stay Fit and Lose Extra Weight

Let's look at 7 Yoga Poses To Achieve An Improved Body. These days, more and more people are getting conscious about their health.

Yoga, as an exercise contributes greatly to

weight loss and an improved overall well-being. It may not burn as many calories compared to traditional exercises. Still, it can help you shed those extra pounds. On the other hand, the technique or routine you're also practicing provides help in the number of calories you'll burn.

If you have gained extra weight over the holidays and wants to shed those off without having to go to the gym or perform vigorous workouts, then it is the perfect time for Yoga. Yoga can also reduce cravings and cut back on our body's ability to deposit fat, it promotes relaxation, and lower our Cortisol levels. Other favorable effects of yoga also include mental gain; you will find yourself paying attention to your body and be fully aware of your changes, both mentally and physically.

Research shows that people have a bad habit of deceiving ourselves of how much they really eat. However, when you practice yoga and achieve self-realization, you would come to understand yourself more especially your manner of eating. Studies show that people often overeat due to boredom or emotional neediness especially when stressed. By knowing this, you could assess yourself, and since you're aware, your eating habits will change. Yoga practice requires movement such as bending, stretching, and meditation which encourages the desire to eat healthily. Not to mention that as a yoga practitioner, you have to follow the Yogi diet. So instead of eating chips or processed foods rich in chemicals or trans fatty acids, you'll crave for fruits and vegetables which are not only food for the body but food for the mind and spirit.

One more wonder that Yoga does to a person is that it'll help you achieve a better self-image and make you feel good about it. That feeling of happiness will then turn into a motivation to be more interested in continuing this practice.

There are plenty of Yoga poses that you can do, and here are the seven poses to help you lose those unwanted pounds. You may already be familiar with it since we covered it the previous chapter.

Vrksasana - Tree Pose

The tree pose is a great standing balance exercise to finish a weight loss yoga flow because your body is expected to be already quite warm and will be in its calorie burning state. The act of balancing takes a tremendous amount of strength, something that most people often don't realize. Every muscle in your body works together to stand in a difficult balancing position. The more your muscles cooperate and move, the better the effect would be.

Since we haven't described this pose, we'll discuss it here.

- Starting with the mountain pose, stand tall and straight with your arms by your sides.
- Bend your right knee lifting your foot off the ground while balancing on just your left foot. Place the bottom of your right foot on your left leg up near your groin.
- Keep your left leg straight and balance your weight on your left leg
- Take a breath and slowly move your arms over your head and bring your hands together in a praying position.
- To help maintain your balance look at a distant object.
- Make sure that your spine is straight. Your entire body should be tight. Relax the body and breath deeply. Hold this pose for at least 30 seconds.

- Slowly lower your hands bringing them in front of your chest as you continue to breathe deeply.
- Now gently lower your arms to your sides and slowly lower your right leg to the floor.
- Complete the pose in the mountain position.
- Now repeat the pose but stand on your right leg.

Veerabhadrasana – Warrior Pose

The warrior poses exercises your legs, thighs, back, and arms. It aids in improving blood circulation, respiration and energizes the entire body. Aside from that, it develops concentration, balance, and groundedness. There are three types of warrior pose: Warrior poses 1, 2 and 3. Each pose has different benefits which include physically, mentally and emotionally benefits. The warrior pose #3 is the best pose for weight loss. It is another pose that involves a fair amount of practice. It takes a lot of core, back and leg strength as well as balance.

Trikonasana - Triangular pose

The triangular pose stretches and strengthens legs, muscles around the knee, ankle joints, hips, groin muscles, hamstrings, calves, shoulders, chest, and spine. Moreover, Triangle pose engages every part of the body and the core. It also opens the hips, shoulders, chest and shoulders

This pose needs to be done properly and consistently to To ensure the superior effect of this pose. If not, it will not provide wanted results.

Purvottanasana - Upward plank

Doing a plank is not as easy as it may seem, even in gym workouts. In as much as it offers effective outcome in other physical activities, it does the same with Yoga. It may be a bit difficult to crack towards the start but the results that this pose produce will leave you much satisfied. This works on your back, shoulders, arms, spine, and wrists and strengthens muscles. It works for the respiratory system too. And it is also excellent in working your legs, inner thigh muscles as wells as hips, mainly targeting the core of your body.

Here's how to do it:

- Sit straight with your legs bent. Lay your hands several inches behind your hips with your finger pointing forward towards your feet. Bend your knees and put your feet on the floor hip-width distance apart.

- As you exhale, push through your hands and feet to mount your hips to the same level as your shoulders then straighten your arms.
- Engage your core muscles as you gradually straighten one leg at a time and point your toes. Vigorously engage your pelvic floor and hoist your hips as high as you can. Keep your legs vigorous and your glutes firm.
- Lie down on your back and lift your chest. Slowly, being mindful of your neck, let your head hang back behind you.
- Hold that pose for up to 30 seconds, then gradually sit back down

Setu Bandha Sarvangasana – Bridge Pose

This pose is one of the most versatile belly exercises; it stretches the spinal cord, neck, thighs, and the hip flexors. By toning the muscles around the spine, this pose will help eliminate unwanted fat around the tummy area. It unfolds the middle and upper part of your spine and inscribes the important alignment systems in your lower body. It also increases the tonicity of the arm and leg muscles helps in digestion and stimulates the thyroid glands and kidneys. It is also great for toning the thighs and abs, as well as strengthening the shoulders.

Utkatasana – Chair Pose

This strengthening posture targets your buttocks and thighs. It also works on your core, back, arms and calf muscles, glutes, hips, back and chest along with the ankle and knee muscles. It's a great pose for overall strength. However, this pose should be avoided if you have a knee or back injury. You may feel pain in your legs for the first couple of days when you practice it. However doing this pose regularly will help you gain flexibility and the pain will vanish.

Chapter 7: A Step Forward to A Happier Life

What does true happiness mean to you? Is it possessing the things you've always wanted? A successful career in your chosen field? Being with the people you love most? Or simply rubbing the belly of your dog or cat? Each and every one of us has our own concept of what happiness truly means.

All of us wants to be happy and to feel joy in our lives. However, the challenges that we encounter along the way and the burdens we carry on our shoulders most of the times make it tough to achieve. As we continue our journey on this planet, these things are inevitable. We just have to think that the harder the situation is, the stronger we become – and mold into a better human being. Yes, it may be easier said than done, but your mentality changes the way you look and react. The universe is like a magnet, if your thoughts are filled with positivity, then good things often come your way, but if one is negativity, then a sequence of unfavorable turnouts can emerge through the surface. It sounds cliché, but it would be best if you ponder that the glass is always half full —meaning, start being an optimist. This way, you'll be able to attract encouraging circumstances to your life, and it may also be a gift you could bestow upon others.

Mandy Hale once said that "Happiness is letting go of what you think your life is supposed to look like and celebrating it for everything that it is." This is a brilliant and inspiring quote to live by. There's that point in our lives where we think that we've hit rock bottom, and it urges us to surrender. We tend to punish ourselves for the mistakes and failures we have made in the past. Hence we forget to appreciate what's happening now. The visions that we have set for our lives to become may not always become a reality. Letting go is not easy all the time, but the key to it is acceptance and hardcore optimism. We have to accept that there are things that we can't change especially the ones that already belong to history, but you can certainly learn from it

There are a lot of books, blogs and personal experiences that could help inspire you to stay positive. Your everyday experiences can be used as lessons. Still, it's necessary to look at the world in a brighter perspective. Be with people who inspires you to bring out your best and never let one failure define who you are. Others may not see the great person you are. Just move on with your life and let them be.

Living a healthy lifestyle also helps you to feel good, and when you feel good inside, your aura oozes with radiance. Live life to the fullest and never let time pass you by without doing anything for yourself. You deserve a break from all the hate and negativity. Did you know that a 30-minute morning exercise can boost your mood for the entire day? Yes, you read that right. Research has shown that moving your body before going to work, school or even staying at home can help you set a feel-good spirit throughout the day. It'll jump start your day to make your more productive in everything you do. Exercise not because other people tell you to do so, but because you want to better yourself. As you move your bones and muscles, shift your thoughts and be as enthusiastic as you are.

A step forward to a healthier life can be challenging, but as you continue to walk the extra mile, you'll find it worth it in the end. In the long run, it will get easier, and you'll feel lighter. Don't ever underestimate your capabilities to make a change and stand up for what true happiness means.

Yoga and You: 5 S' That'll Surprise You And Turn Your Life Around

Leading a healthy life can mean a happy life. Getting yourself moving can provide you with the energy that you need every day. We have mentioned previously that there are a lot of exercises you can do to help achieve a healthier lifestyle and one of which is Yoga.

Stress in just one of the major factors that contribute to an unhappy life. When you are stressed, you can easily get irritated. Stress can make you extermly angry or frustrated. It can affect your productivity at work and your mood inside your household. Almost everything around you is affected. Let me reiterate that Yoga can help reduce stress levels which are significant.

Considering Yoga as part of your life can make a huge impact on how to perceive and interpret the things that are happening around you. Yoga's benefits to a happier life can be more surprising than you think. Ultimately, here are five advantages Yoga can add to your welfare.

1. **Self-Esteem**

Yoga helps you become fit. When you feel

good about how you look, self-esteem and confidence start to build. With exercises and routines, you'll be fully aware of what you're capable of and determine your limitations. Having self-esteem builds a personality with little fear. It allows you to get rid of negativity that lurks inside your head and helps you will feel peacefulness, and strength.

The meditation exercises of yoga can help you understand that you are whom you are. You need to live with yourself. You can improve yourself, and your body. However you must live with yourself. This is the concept that limitations are not downfalls, but simply who and what you are. Once you have accepted the things that you can and can't do, your self-confidence will intensify.

It can also strengthen your mind to believe in yourself and what you are capable of. No matter what challenge comes your way, you will be confident enough to face it. Having self-confidence can make you care less of what other people think about you

2. Soulful Existence

Yoga helps fight the signs of stress and

moderate its levels. Aside from that, its meditation exercises allow you to reach the inner cores of your mind and spirit. You'll learn how to live in the moment and appreciate the true meaning of your life.

Yoga allows you to recognize the good things and keep you mindful of what's happening around you. It gives you the benefit of seeing your positive value, hence, transforms you into a rejuvenated and recharged person – a better version of yourself. Your mind and approach to life may gain some flexibility as well.

Holistic healing can change a person, and it will certainly provide you a happier life. It encourages you to do, think and speak good things with people that surround you. Given this, you allow goodness to enter your life, thus, generously give portions of it to your fellow men. Forgiving easily, letting go of futile stuff that doesn't matter. Meaning, you're just not merely living to survive, but you exist with greater sense. You're living a higher purpose in this world, and you would feel the fulfillment from within knowing that you have done the right thing.

3. **Standpoint**

Mindfulness With Yoga

Meditation and breathing exercises of Yoga work wonder on your mind, body and spirit – a holistic healing. This allows better outlook and understanding of things. Feeling good inside can calm and relax your mind. This can make room for positive things to happen. It allows your mind to retreat from your hectic lifestyle.

Yoga attracts positivity helping you to see the brighter side of life no matter how obscure the road may be. It cleanses your mind from negative thoughts and makes out the journey's right destination as well as the way leading to it. Optimistic people tend to have favorable views towards the world. Being positive can help people to be more productive, be brighter, and keep that 'feel good' vibe which can influence a good physical and mental health.

It's fulfilling to know that you are looking at the world in a different point of view. You're not only helping yourself but others as well. You can be their candle in the night, a guide that leads to them through the dark. A positive standpoint can lift you higher, and you'll be surprised how much you can achieve. Plus, it can kindle the spirit within you to never surrender and just focus on your goal.

4. Success

When you accomplish a task or a goal, normally, you call it a success, right? And it makes you happy knowing that you did your best to do it. Success has many forms, and it depends on how you perceive it to be. However, no matter what success means to you, Yoga will be there to guide you.

The other S advantages that we have mentioned previously are interconnected to each other, especially to success. When you have self-esteem, positive standpoint and soulful existence, you are most likely to succeed in life. Why? It is because you can handle stress better and you are more enthusiastic in everything you do. Yoga can help you focus on what's important and disregard negative thoughts as you move along. You possess patience on your task because you have a calm and relaxed mind. Yoga exercises work its magic in building your body to be ready for your life's journey.

Yoga Meditation exercise is all about relaxing a busy mind, directing you to live and experience each moment to the fullest. So, once you achieve something, even how simple it is, the joy you can feel deep in your heart is indescribable. Especially if you lifted other people along in your success. Seeing them happy and celebrating your success with them, that's more success than you could ever hope for – that's called life fulfillment.

5. Sex

Yes, you read it right. Yoga can help you achieve a better and happier sex life. Aside from the physical improvement, Yoga exercises also help the release of endorphins, which are called the "feel-good" hormones of our body, allowing us to be happy, and feel less pain. Studies have shown that Yoga can lowers stress levels. This can make you in the mood more often and less likely to argue with your significant other. Also, yoga involves engaging and drawing up the muscles of the pelvic area, which strengthens the muscles that play an integral role in sex. It is clear that yoga can boost athletic performance, but Yoga also helps when it comes to making love. Some studies have indicated that Yoga exercise can also be advantageous when it comes to making act of love making more satisfying. Its physical benefits sanction you to be more flexible in bed, especially in performing different sexual positions. The outcome will be an increase in sexual desire as well as sexual gratification. Additionally, it is believed that by marginally contracting the coccygeal pub muscles can heighten arousal and amend sexual performance. All this is possible by a remote muscle contraction phenomenon that composes an energetic seal that locks breath in our body, which then carries circulation and information to the pelvic region.

Moreover, regular practice helps to strengthen, lengthen and tone your body, and all of these will make you feel better about yourself. Thus, it will boost your self-confidence. that will help you feel more sexy and comfortable with another body beside you.

Life

There are a lot of reasons to celebrate life and be happy with what is happening at present. There may be bumps in the road, but the path will never change. You just have to keep going and don't lose yourself along the way. Live life as it is, and as long as you embody the teachings of Yoga, you should always expect the unexpected. For you'll never know when another surprise shall arrive at the right moment. Despite the fact that some of the things we want are insatiable, our overall being can still be satisfied if holistic healing has taken its toll and make us aware of the things that truly matter in this world – Things that are more than what meets the naked eye.

Techniques To Achieve Inner Peace

Inner peace probably is the most difficult condition to achieve. No matter how hard we try most of the time, a lot of the time we don't pay attention to events or situations that occur around us. The intensity of the situation can hurt us, and we tend to react to it in an adverse manner. Sometimes, it's easier to convince ourselves that we have peace and that what others think about us is none of our business, yet, subconsciously, we think about it. It's like we're pretending to make the situation better, or so it seems, but the fact is, it makes it even harder to overcome.

With very high respect to Buddha, I recalled one of his teachings about inner peace which says, "Inner peace begins the moment you choose not to allow another person or event to control your emotions." Just like happiness, inner peace is also a matter of choice. Convincing ourselves to believe something that is not entirely true can cause emotional stress, without even knowing it. Sometimes, when things are unbearable, instead of letting ourselves control the situation, it turns out that the situation controls us. It takes us around, and if things get bad, then we can get caught up in the moment without realizing that we no longer have control over our own emotions.

This is where Yoga can work its magic. It's holistic healing that allows us to reach the far corners of our core, to know the real us – who we really are and what we're capable of. We were born to be unique, and we hold enigmatic power over our mind if we only knew about it.

Inner peace chases a person who trains with a purpose in mind. It is more than just being true to yourself; you have to find the truth in order, to be honest with everyone. If you have a feeling of guilt, insecurity, or any other inferior emotions, you have to unravel the deeper truth of what they are, and why they are the way they are. Once you find the answer and accept it, it is only then you can finally be free from the chains that stop you from achieving relief or inner peace.

Remember in the movie, Kung Fu Panda 2, where Po's mission was to find inner peace? He was distracted all along and was confused about who he really is. Thus, he loses his way. The moment when he stopped fighting his own memories and just let it all flow as he does meditation, he was able to find out all the answers to his questions. In the end, he found his true identity, purpose and who he was meant to be – he unlocked the doors of inner peace. Just like him, you have to dig deeper to find what you're looking for. The only person standing between you and inner peace is you.

Years of Yoga practice can be of great benefit to you in achieving inner peace, here are techniques you can learn from.

Meditation Of The Soul: Rediscover Yourself

As we grow wiser and older, the number of challenges we stumble upon are countless. During the battles that we face to survive and succeed, most of the times we lose ourselves, and we become a different person. The hectic lifestyle also affects the quality of person we develop into. In time, we drift further from our true self, just like a caged animal, petrified and detached from ourselves.

You deserve better, though. Take time to relax, breathe and assess yourself. Yoga meditation exercises allow you to travel deep into the past. Bring the truth out of your inner self, let go of judgments and competition with others. Rediscover your strengths and find the beauty within you. The calm that a yoga practice brings helps rid the chaos, frustration, and exhaustion that commonly fills the mind.

Every time you dive into the zone of your true self, the deeper you'll understand your purpose. You'll come to realize that you're more than what you thought you're capable of. Negative criticisms from people around you will not matter anymore.

You may find yourself less susceptible in life situations. In addition, rediscovering yourself will unfold your true balance and no matter how hard life gets. Still, you're able to maintain a positive attitude. Your productivity will increase, the way you treat other people will greatly improve, you'll be happier, and your appreciation of simple yet meaningful things will be nourishing to the soul.

Defy Age and Start A New Chapter Of Life

Age is just a number and youth is a state of mind. Science confirmed that Yoga offers age-defying benefits. Yoga exercises help improve our memory and mental intelligence. All powerful components to maintain a positive quality of life as we age. Recent clinical studies show that daily practice fosters a true sense of calm and compassion, and cultivates a deep inner shift in our life perspective, creating renewed energy to live life more fully, and with genuine enjoyment.

Given the positive effects of Yoga in defying or even reversing the effects of aging, it's never too late to start a new life. Regardless of your age, if your mind is rejuvenated by Yoga, your journey to find inner peace can commence anytime. Yoga practice will provide you true self-realization and inner peace as you age in years, but not in the state of your mind.

As we age, we gain more knowledge and acquire the wisdom of the past. But, does it then follow that we already have discovered who we are? Or is the past still haunting you at such age? Well, you better start your journey in discovering inner peace now. Make peace with your past and do the things as you wish without any regrets. Let go of your fear and let your true self-guide you towards the new chapter of your life – a better tale of who you really are despite your age.

Where the Mind Goes, The Body Will Follow (Transform Your Mind)

Have you ever experienced that, your body wants to do something or be anywhere, but when your brain tells you otherwise, you just end up doing nothing? Well, it's a simple representation of how powerful your mind is. If you continue to let your negative or idle thoughts take control of your entire body, then you're just wasting your life. You'll never find peace of mind because someday, one way or another, your greatest enemy will be regret.

No matter how hard you try to move on, at the back of your mind, still regret speaks a loud voice, telling you that you should have done what you should when you had the chance. Let Yoga be your instrument in transforming your mind and let it take your body to great places.

Meditation exercises that Yoga offer will allow you to realize the true power of your mind – where the mind goes, the body will follow. Your positive, uplifting thoughts shall encourage your inner self to do what you want and what you needed. It'll transform your mind to let go of fear and other negative emotions and utilize your rejuvenated self's capability to achieve things.

Having Less Means Having More

There are times in our lives when we have almost everything that we wanted, yet, there's that emptiness inside. It's because it's not what you really need. Those things are what you want. As long as you seek happiness in material things, you would never feel contented and happy. In as much as you disregard the value of simple things or gestures, that hole inside your will never be filled. The key here is, you have to look beyond what you see. The fewer things you posse, the more internal satisfaction you have, given that, you can get a hold of what's really important.

Yoga exercises, as what we have mentioned previously. Provides holistic healing. It rejuvenates and transforms you into a better person with a positive way of thinking. As you meditate, your mind get rids of all the refineries, the unnecessary things that you possess, and you only have you – the true you. From there, you realize that extravagant material objects won't satisfy your need. Love, family, a good job, a nice house and good friends would mean a lot. You may not have a fancy car; you have a whole lot more. Making memories is much important than making money to be rich. In the end, you can't buy happiness or inner peace. You may even lose the people you love if you don't realize it until it's too late.

Conclusion

Congratulations! You have made it to the end of our book, "Mindfulness With Yoga: Stress-Free Life And Inner Peace." We went over a lot so stick around for a quick recap. At this point, you should be a mindfulness, yoga, and meditation master! We went over the benefits, the practices, and many convincing reasons you should be starting today. Here's what we went over:

In the first chapter, we went over what exactly mindfulness is. As you learned, it is the psychological process of bringing attention to both your internal and external experiences. Remember that a lot of us fall into a vicious cycle of feeling bad about certain events, and then feeling bad about feeling bad. So, what was one of the main concepts of mindfulness? That's right! Acceptance! While we are being mindful, we are acknowledging any feelings or thoughts we may be having. As Jon Kabat Zinn said, "Mindfulness meaning paying attention in a particular way; on purpose, in the present moment, and nonjudgmentally.'

The second chapter then introduced

meditation for mindfulness. Here, we learned that meditation is used to help us accept us as we are. What position was it that we suggested for this practice? Sitting! In this same chapter, we followed step by step to cover the three basic aspects of meditation. Do you remember what they were? Body, breath, and thoughts. From here, we introduced the concept of choosing your environment, taking in your environment, practicing your breathing, and finally how to practice working on your thoughts. Remember that when you are new to meditation, you may not get it instantly. The concept isn't about perfection; it's about the practice and making yourself happy!

We then went over yoga and mindfulness in the third chapter. What do you remember from this section? We first want you to remember all of the amazing benefits that you can gain from yoga. First, there were the health benefits like gaining a better immune system, lowering your blood pressure, and increasing your blood circulation. There were also health benefits that experience without your body such as a delayed aging process, a better posture, and even getting better sleep from being so relaxed. If this wasn't enough to convince you, also remember that there are many emotional health benefits to practicing yoga. Being relaxed can help stress reduction, can lower anxiety, and improve your mood, and also helps people gain a better self-acceptance. Last, we introduced you to some of the basic yoga positions to get you started on your path to becoming a yogi. With all of those amazing benefits, we listed, why wouldn't you want to learn and practice yoga.

In our fourth chapter, we quickly covered both mindful-based cognitive therapy as well as mindfulness-based stress reduction. The important aspect to remember from this chapter is the fact that MBCT is used for patients that suffer from major depression disorders. The therapy is an eight-week program used to help depression patients understand what they are going through and then accepting it as it comes. Do you remember how long this was? Right, a two-hour weekly course and then a day long retreat. The psychologist found how being mindful could be beneficial and applied it to this specific disorder but remember that MBSR is also used for a wider range of disorders.

In our fifth chapter, we covered some basic tips to begin mindfulness for beginners. Which one do you remember the most? Remember to keep it simple and take the time to get some mindful meditation in your life. As we learned, a lot of us rush through life and try to get as much done as possible. You do not have to live like the other half do. Remember to take time for yourself and practice on your breathing. The more you practice, the easier mindful meditation will be. Also, LET IT GO! You are going to get distracted. When you sit down to practice, don't be surprised when you keep having thoughts pop into your head. This concept will become easier with more time and more practice. Start with the breathing and then move on to the thoughts. We guarantee that it will be well worth the effort.

In our sixth chapter, we covered the yoga diet. We talked about how the yoga diet does not include meat or junk food. It is made up of lots of fruits and vegetables. We also talked about how the diet affects the body in regards to blood sugar, blood pressure, balance, bone health, sound sleep, immune system, flexibility and posture, stress and weight loss. We also reviewed some yoga poses for weight loss.

In our eighth chapter, we covered a step forward to a happier life. This chapter should still be fresh in your mind. To quickly review we covered: self-esteem, soulful existence, standpoint, success, sex, life, techniques to achieve inner peace, meditation of the soul, defy age, Where the mind Goes the body with follow, less means more.

We hope that you enjoyed our book and that you were able to take away some knowledge about mindfulness with you. By being relaxed, you may find yourself having an easier, and happier life. We hope that by finding mindfulness in your life, you allow the time to practice yoga and meditation. Not only will you reap the benefits of these practices, but also can find yourself applying the skills to your daily lives. We wish you the best of luck on your journey. Live a happy, healthy life.

ABOUT THE AUTHOR

John Francisco has been writing for many years. He was born in California but grew up in the Wisconsin. He has always had an interest in producing informational books and other material. Since 2004 John has lived and worked in or around Chicago, Illinois.